Get to Know
Your Gut

About the Authors

JOAN SAUERS is the author of seven non-fiction books, including *Quick Fixes for Everyday Back Pain*. She suffered from a number of ailments described in this book before finding the right formula to maintain digestive health. Joan has also worked in Hollywood as a script reader and editor for Fox and Zoetrope Studios, has run a film production company in New York, and currently writes and edits television and film screenplays. She lectures in screenwriting at film schools in London, Paris, and Berlin. Born in New York, Joan lives in Sydney with her daughter Ruby.

JOANNA MCMILLAN-PRICE is a nutrition scientist with a BSc (Hons) in Nutrition & Dietetics and on track to complete her PhD soon at The University of Sydney. She is the coauthor of *The Low GI Diet Revolution*, a consultant dietitian to *Slimming* magazine, a regular guest on ABC radio, and lectures on nutrition both in Australia and the UK. Joanna is also a qualified fitness leader and teaches group exercise classes in her "spare" time. Born in Scotland, Joanna emigrated to Australia in 1999 and lives with her family in Sydney.

Get to Know Your Gut

Everything You Wanted to Know about Burping,
Bloating, Candida, Constipation, Food Allergies,
Farting and Poo but Were Afraid to Ask

Joan Sauers
with Joanna McMillan-Price, BSc (Hons)

MARLOWE & COMPANY
NEW YORK

GET TO KNOW YOUR GUT

Everything You Wanted to Know about Burping, Bloating, Candida, Constipation, Food Allergies, Farting and Poo but Were Afraid to Ask

Copyright © 2005 by Joan Sauers

Published by
Marlowe & Company
An Imprint of Avalon Publishing Group Incorporated
245 West 17th Street • 11th floor
New York, NY 10011

AVALON
publishing group incorporated

First published in 2004 as *Gut Reactions* by ABC Books in Australia. This edition published by arrangement.

Library of Congress Cataloging-in-Publication Data
Sauers, Joan, 1953-
Get to know your gut: everyhing you wanted to know about burping, bloating, candida, constipation, food allergies, farting, and poo but were afraid to ask/Joan Sauers, with Joanna McMillan-Price.
p. cm
Includes index.
ISBN 1-56924-370-0
1. Gastrointestinal system--Diseases--Popular works. 2. Digestion--Popular works. 3. Indigestion--Popular works. I. McMillan-Price, Joanna. II. Title.

RC806.S28 2005
616.3'3--dc22
2004065584

9 8 7 6 5 4 3 2 1

Designed by Maria Elias

Printed in Canada

Contents

Introduction   *xiii*

One

Digestion Basics   *1*

The role of the digestive system   2

The digestive system   2

Burping, bloating, and farting   *16*

Stools   *22*

Two

Digestive Disorders   27

Halitosis (bad breath)   *28*

Indigestion and heartburn (reflux)   *30*

Nausea and vomiting   *35*

Gastroenteritis   38

Constipation   47

Hemorrhoids   54

Irritable bowel syndrome (IBS)   55

Ulcers   59

Food allergies, intolerance, and sensitivity   62

Inflammatory bowel disease (colitis and
Crohn's disease)   70

Appendicitis   73

Diverticulitis   74

Gall bladder disease   76

Candida   78

Hirschsprung's disease   82

Colorectal cancer   83

Stomach cancer   86

AIDS   88

Colic   88

Hiatus hernia   90

Leaky gut syndrome   91

Hormonal fluctuations   91

Eating disorders   92

Support groups   93

Three

Food, Supplements, and Digestion   **95**

Make food welcome   97

Foods that can aid digestion   98

Food "accessories"   105

Water   113

Fiber   114

To meat or not to meat?   121

Raw food   123

Supplements   124

Four

Drugs and Digestion   *135*

Antibiotics   *136*

Acid suppressants and antacids   *137*

Antispasmodics and muscle relaxers   *138*

Opioid analgesics   *139*

Alginate   *140*

Laxatives   *140*

Anti-inflammatories   *141*

Antidepressants and tranquillizers   *142*

Nonsteroidal anti-inflammatory drugs
(NSAIDs)   *143*

Lipase inhibitors   *144*

Marijuana   *144*

Smoking   *145*

Five

Stress and Digestion   147

Visualization   149

Meditation   150

Aromatherapy   152

Medication   153

Easy ways to stress less   154

Six

Practitioners, Tests,
and Digestive Disorders   157

Diagnostic tests   159

Gastroenterology   166

Nutritional science   167

Complementary therapies   168

Seven

Exercising for Digestion   *185*

    Walking and running   *185*

    Yoga   *186*

    Pilates   *187*

    Abdominal workouts   *188*

Eight

The Bottom Line   *191*

    Acknowledgments   *193*

    Index   *195*

Let food be thy medicine and thy medicine be thy food.
—Hippocrates

Introduction

*D*igesting food is as basic to human survival as breathing air. And yet all too often our digestive systems seem to fail us. Indigestion, heartburn, nausea, ulcers, constipation, diarrhea, and many more serious conditions commonly occur in developed countries like the United States where these things shouldn't be on the rise. But they are.

One reason for this is that most of us still don't really understand how our guts work and what we could be doing to help them work better. Another reason is that some of the medical establishment have been slow to embrace the idea of nutritional therapy for digestive disorders, and sometimes the conventional treatment hasn't helped.

But perhaps the biggest reason is that many of us have simply learned to live with symptoms like bad breath or hemorrhoids, because they don't seem all that serious.

This is unacceptable. It's time that we took responsibility for our digestive health. Now there are no more excuses.

There have been huge leaps forward in the understanding of digestive diseases that are gradually filtering down to street level. But one problem is that a lot of the information is so technical—and *conflicting!*—that it's easier to keep doing what we're doing, even if it's not good for us. Another problem is that people (over the age of five) can be a little shy talking about things like burping, farting, and bowel movements.

But shyness when it comes to our health can be dangerous. Avoiding issues that make us uncomfortable can allow conditions to worsen. To quote the American Cancer Society slogan, "Don't die of embarrassment."

What this book is about is making things easier to understand and hopefully easier to talk about and then deal with. Your digestive health is in your hands, and no amount of doctors and specialists and nutritionists can cure what's wrong with your gut *without your help.*

Digestion Basics *One*

When we talk about the gut, we're just trying to be friendly and keep it simple. But the digestive system is actually a lot more than just your intestines.

It's really important to think of your body as a working whole rather than a grab bag of individual parts. You are a mini-ecosystem where everything is interconnected and inter-dependent. And we don't just mean your kneebone's connected to your thighbone. We mean that what you see, what you feel, how you think, what you eat, how you move, how you breathe—virtually everything that you do—affects you physically as a whole. And everything that affects you physically as a whole affects your digestion.

The role of the digestive system

Essentially, the digestive system is supposed to take in fuel in the form of food, which it then breaks down so that we can absorb the usable nutrients and then expel what we don't need. It sounds so easy, and yet there are so many stages and processes involved that it gets very complex very quickly. It will help if you can picture what happens, so we'll give you a little tour of the digestive labyrinth.

The digestive system

The digestive system is a network of organs, glands, muscles, nerves, and chemicals that interacts with the circulatory, lymphatic, and musculoskeletal systems, as well as the brain. Sound complicated? It is. But for now we'll focus on the gastrointestinal tract (also known as the GIT—not to be confused with the *gut*, which just means your intestines), which you've probably seen illustrated in one of those attractive wall charts at the doctor's office.

The importance of the GIT can be gauged by the fact that it has the largest blood supply in the body as well as a huge nerve system, comparable in the number of nerves to the spinal cord. One of the most important—the vagus

The Long and Winding Road: your gastrointestinal tract (GIT)

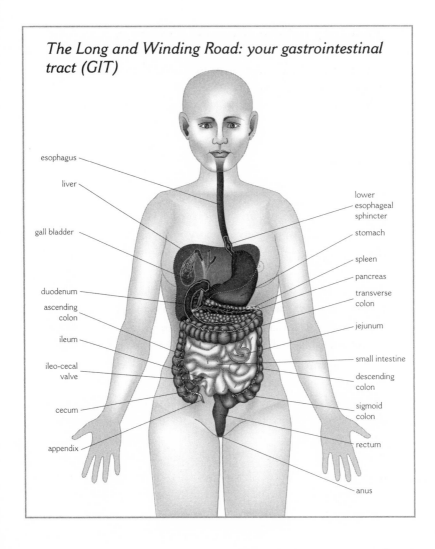

esophagus

liver

gall bladder

duodenum

ascending colon

ileum

ileo-cecal valve

cecum

appendix

lower esophageal sphincter

stomach

spleen

pancreas

transverse colon

jejunum

small intestine

descending colon

sigmoid colon

rectum

anus

nerve—carries messages back and forth between the brain and the digestive tract constantly, which is how emotions like depression, fear, joy, and being pissed off at your boss can influence digestion.

The senses

You might think the digestive road starts with the mouth, but it actually starts elsewhere. If you think about your favorite food, especially when you're hungry, your mouth will start to water. That's a chemical response triggered by your brain. So it started in your mind. Or you might not be thinking about food, but you walk past a nice Italian restaurant where they're cooking spaghetti sauce and as you inhale the fragrance your mouth starts to water. In this case, it started in your nose. Or maybe you just sit down to dinner and look at the beautiful meal of sushi your boyfriend just prepared (okay, he probably got it take-out) and your mouth starts to water. So the process started with your eyes. In all these cases, the digestive process actually began before food passed your lips. So digestion is a multi-sensory experience.

Saliva

Why do our mouths fill with saliva as we anticipate food? Because we need it to start the digestive process. While our saliva is about 99.5 percent water, the rest is made up of useful enzymes, salts, and minerals that we need to perform a variety of jobs. The enzymes start the job of breaking down carbohydrates, including sugars and starch, and also kill bacteria that may be lurking in the food. The salts and minerals are for pH (acidity) balance, and there's even something in there to make the food slippery so you can swallow it easily. Saliva is a marvelous cocktail. Even when you're not eating you continue to produce it in small amounts to keep your mouth and teeth clean and prevent plaque build-up. If you don't produce enough saliva, you might have a dry mouth, bad teeth, and a hard time swallowing.

The tongue

We're born with about 10,000 taste buds on our tongues, although many can become useless by adulthood, especially if we smoke. But when they're working, each taste bud contains nerves that send information to our brains about the food we're eating, which then experience the information as taste. Different taste buds are sensitive to different tastes—sweet at the tip of the tongue, salty in the middle, sour on the sides, bitter at the back. All this information triggers the release of digestive juices in the stomach, which is now getting as excited as your mouth was when you first got a whiff of that spaghetti sauce.

Taste buds also come in different sizes, so don't panic if you notice that you have lumps arranged in a V shape at the back of your tongue. They're just taste buds, and don't indicate any sort of disorder.

Chewing and the teeth

Our teeth have the very important job of chopping and grinding food, and while this may seem to be an easy, basic function, almost all of us don't chew our food enough! The act of chewing tells your brain that food is coming so it can increase the flow of digestive juice in the stomach. If you don't chew enough there won't be enough digestive juice in the stomach to break the food down properly. Also, if food goes down in big chunks it can end up in the lower bowel where it feeds bacteria and makes gas. So bloating and flatulence can be caused by simply not chewing thoroughly.

What's thoroughly? Thoroughly is turning food into a soft paste before you swallow. We mean you should *really* pulverize it. This will come as a shock to the many people who approach meals like vacuum cleaners. (You know who you are!) The trick is to eat *slowly*. Food is not meant to be inhaled. If you rush through a meal you can't possibly be chewing enough. There are a few tricks, like taking smaller bites than you normally would, and even putting your fork and knife down in between bites so you're not eating like an industrial vacuum on high speed. Also, it will help if you don't talk with your mouth full, which is some people's only form of multi-tasking. Sad but true. And don't try the old shortcut of drinking lots of fluids while you eat to wash the big chunks down. The fluid will only make matters worse once the un-mashed food gets to your stomach.

A note about chewing gum. Don't do it unless you're about to eat, because it makes the digestive juice (full of acid) start flowing, and some practitioners suggest that if your stomach's empty the acid can produce gas and may irritate your stomach lining, causing possible long-term damage. Bloating can also be caused by swallowing extra air as you chew. And frankly, it's a pretty unattractive thing to do.

Of course all this chewing can only be done properly with a healthy set of teeth. If your teeth are missing, falling out, ground down, or your gums are diseased, it's unlikely that you're chewing food as well as you could. And you need to chew well to get food into the shape it needs to be for the rest of the digestive tract to handle it. Unless you want to live off soup for the rest of your life. And by the way, bad teeth are unattractive too.

So follow the basic rules for maintaining dental health. Brush your teeth regularly, ideally after every meal. Ditto flossing. A lot of people still haven't been convinced by dentists or their accompanying heart-stopping bills that flossing is as essential as brushing. The principle is simple: food that gets caught between the teeth will gradually contribute to cavities that will eventually cause you to lose the teeth. Saliva can only do so much in terms of keeping your mouth clean. It can't get to material that's wedged too deeply.

If you grind your teeth, as so many of us do, your teeth may be suffering the effects. Long-term grinding can blunt or flatten teeth, especially the molars, which we need to really pulverize our food. Your dentist will be able to recommend a course of action to solve the problem, and these days you have a wide variety of options. You may be fitted with a splint, or plate, which slips onto your upper teeth like a boxer's mouth guard, but slimmer. Wearing this while sleeping can stop you from grinding, and also prevent the nasty side-effects like TMJ (temporomandibular joint disorder), jaw clicking, headaches, and the dreadful noise of grinding that can often keep others awake.

Instead of a splint, your dentist might suggest having small extensions added to your teeth, which look just like the real thing and can actually prevent you from grinding by creating tiny lifts and barriers. These will also make chewing easier and therefore aid digestion.

Of course a lot of grinding is caused by stress, so stress management, which we'll discuss later, is another option to consider when trying to maintain dental and digestive health.

The esophagus

Once your food is wellchewed (hopefully), your tongue maneuvers it to the back of your throat where it enters the muscular tube leading to the stomach called the esophagus. The wave-like movement of food through the esophagus is called peristalsis, an action that will be repeated at later stages along the digestive tract. While swallowing is a conscious movement, peristalsis through the GIT is unconscious or autonomic.

At the bottom of the esophagus, food then passes into the stomach through a muscular one-way valve called the lower esophageal sphincter. This sphincter is very useful, as it prevents food from flowing back into the esophagus when you lie flat or even hang upside down. Of course sometimes, especially after some sophisticated social encounter like boys' night out or an office Christmas party, food—and booze— will come up anyway and you will experience reverse peristalsis, also known as puking, which will be addressed later at greater length.

The stomach

The stomach is an organ made of muscle, about the size of a grapefruit, shaped like a fat letter "j." When food arrives, there should already be enough digestive juice there to take care of it. Stomach "juice" is actually another digestive cocktail, this time made up of enzymes and hydrochloric acid. The acid is strong—not quite as powerful as the drool from the creatures in the movie *Alien*, but still strong. If you plopped a few drops of your own stomach acid on your skin it would gradually burn through to the bone. Luckily you have a 1-inch thick mucous-coated lining that protects the stomach wall from being broken down by your own acid. The job of hydrochloric acid is to kill harmful bacteria and micro-organisms that still might be lingering in the food and also help break down proteins.

But it isn't just a chemical process that takes place in the stomach. The muscles of your stomach actually churn and crush the food, although you usually don't feel this because you don't have as many sensory nerves in the stomach as in your skin or other parts of the body. Of course every once in a while you *can* feel stomach movement, which is not a bad thing; in fact it's nice to know it's there doing its job.

Not many nutrients are absorbed through the stomach wall, but drugs like alcohol and aspirin do penetrate and get straight through to the bloodstream. That's why food sits in your stomach for hours, but you can feel the effects of a shot of vodka almost instantly. When it comes to food, carbohydrates get broken down first and then proteins, and fats sit there the longest, up to about four hours. That's why, after you have a fatty meal, you feel full for a long time: you are! And that's why they say that after Chinese food you're hungry again in an hour; most Chinese food is low in fat compared to fried chicken and mashed potatoes with gravy. The thing to understand is that you're not really hungry again—it's just that you're not overly full, which is what too many people brought up on a Western diet believe is the right way to feel after a meal.

Only once your stomach is completely empty will you start to feel hungry again, and your digestive juice will build up to workable levels. That's why it's a really good idea to eat only when you're hungry, and not just for pleasure. If you add new food to half-digested food already in your stomach, your digestive juice will be overwhelmed and you will inadequately digest what's there. But of course every once in a while (especially on a hot day at the beach) you're allowed to treat yourself to an ice-cream cone, even though you just had lunch. The first rule of good health (and mental stability) is "everything in moderation, including moderation."

The small intestine

After it's been through your own personal food processor, food is then pushed by the stomach muscles through another valve called the pylorus into the duodenum, which makes up the first inch or so of the small intestine. At this point, food is called chyme (pronounced *kime*). Collectively, the small intestine and large intestine are also known as the bowel.

The duodenum is where other organs really start collaborating with the digestive tract to break things down. (So remember the delicate balance of that ecosystem.) Chyme is very acidic, and would damage the duodenum if not for the buffering effect of the alkaline juice secreted from the pancreas and gall bladder.

The pancreas not only helps neutralize acid, but also produces enzymes that further digest carbohydrates, fats, and proteins. The gall bladder also contributes by storing and delivering bile that was produced in the liver and helps to break down fats. Later on, from the bloodstream, the liver will filter through nutrients and either store them or send them where they're needed in the body.

The stuff in your digestive tract is now an amazing cocktail of chemicals with molecules small enough to cross the intestinal wall and be absorbed into the bloodstream and lymphatic vessels. Most nutrients are absorbed in the duodenum, but some get through further along. Let's hope you chewed thoroughly so no big chunks are floating around at this point, unable to be assimilated.

The small intestine is between nineteen and twenty-one feet long and about an inch in diameter, winding its way back and forth, eventually heading south. But the really exciting thing about it is that its walls are lined with a kind of organic shag carpeting, and each tiny projection is called a villus.

The villi are covered in microscopic microvilli and there are from 3,000 to 6,000 microvilli on each cell! It's through the microvilli that you absorb nutrients. Together, the folds, villi, and microvilli increase the surface area of your small intestine so that it's 600 times greater than it would be if your intestinal tract were just a tube. Which means that your small intestine has the approximate surface area of somewhere between a tennis court and a football field.

A healthy intestinal lining absorbs good nutrients but blocks bad things like unfriendly bugs and allergens with its own immune system. Eighty percent of your lymph nodes, where white blood cells are made, are positioned around the intestinal tract to keep bad news out. And as long as you're healthy, the cells of your intestinal lining are replaced every three to six days—*very* fast compared to the rest of the body—so that this filtering system stays efficient.

The other thing that's happening in your small intestine is peristalsis—the wave-like contraction and relaxation of the intestinal muscles that keeps the chyme moving along. When things are working properly, you have around twelve of these waves per minute.

The colon or large intestine

The small intestine ends at another one-way junction called the ileocecal valve, which allows the flow of the remaining chyme into the colon. The colon, or large intestine, is about five to six and a half feet long and two and a half to three and a half inches in diameter. It's shaped like an upside-down "U," rising up on the right (the ascending colon) then going across (the transverse colon) and heading down (the descending colon) on the left to the rectum.

The colon isn't really designed to absorb food, and by the time chyme gets there most digestion has occurred, although water and some nutrients do cross the colon wall. At this point most of what's left is waste, which is merely stored until it can be eliminated. When you're ready to eliminate it, waste goes into the rectum and out through the anus. It's important

The surface area of your small intestine . . .
Tennis anyone?

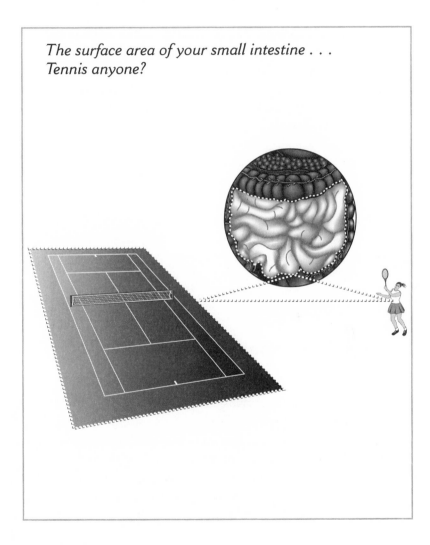

not to store things for too long, and a whole host of disorders can arise from not keeping all parts of the bowel moving. It shouldn't take food more than a day or so to get from mouth to motion, but in "developed" countries like the United States and Australia where most of us favor Western-style diets, it takes, on the average, two to four days. Or longer. This is mostly due to diet and lifestyle.

If you're curious about how long it takes to travel your inner road, swallow a few spoonfuls of cooked corn kernels and see when they appear in your stools. If it's longer than thirty or forty hours, your bowel is too sluggish and you should think about things like more fiber, more water, and more exercise. Some people never see the corn again! A scary thought. But more on that later.

Burping, bloating, and farting

While gas will be mentioned later in connection with various digestive disorders, a certain amount of it is also a totally normal by-product of the digestive process. And it holds such an important place in the scheme of gut-related things that it demands its own section. And although a foolish few may deny it, everybody does it. At both ends.

The average person unleashes anywhere from 400 milliliters to 2,400 milliliters of flatus, or bowel gas, per day. That's around seven farts from the average woman, and 14 from the average guy. It only *seems* like 10 times that much. The figures on burps were unavailable at the time of publication. So where does all that gas come from?

A lot of gas comes from swallowing air when we talk and when we eat, especially if we do these things too fast or at the same time. People who breathe through their mouths, including snorers and those with blocked sinuses, will ingest a lot of air. We also swallow even more air when we drink than when we eat, especially drinking through a straw, or from a can or bottle. And if what's in the bottle has bubbles, look out. Dentures that don't fit quite right can also make you swallow excess air. Yet another reason to take care of your teeth!

Most swallowed air comes up through burping, although some carries through to the colon where it's either reabsorbed or expelled through farting.

But swallowed air is only half (or less) of the story of gas. At least half of our gas we make ourselves when bacteria in the colon breaks down what is left of the food we've eaten. And different foods produce different effects, in terms of both volume and fragrance. Some of the foods that are particularly renowned for producing intestinal gas are: beans (but like other foods that are high in fiber, they cause less smell than meats and spices), Jerusalem artichokes, many Asian spices, fatty foods,

It's a long way to the bottom if you wanna look at it that way!

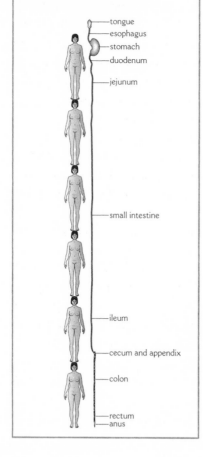

tongue
esophagus
stomach
duodenum
jejunum

small intestine

ileum

cecum and appendix

colon

rectum
anus

unripe bananas, eggs (in quantity), cabbage, cauliflower, broccoli, Brussels sprouts, eggplant, meat, mushrooms, turnips, fennel, poppy and sunflower seeds, onions, garlic, and leeks. Excessive sugar may also contribute to the production of gas in the colon. Beans will produce less gas if you soak them for a day and a half before you cook them, and though it may seem strange, broccoli, Brussels sprouts, cabbage, cauliflower, and turnips will produce less gas the *less* you cook them.

But don't avoid high-fiber vegetables and legumes just because they produce gas. The trick is too add these foods gradually to your diet and your body will accommodate them without too many fireworks. Eventually you'll be no more gassy than you were before you started eating beans. Sorbitol causes gas big time, and while it's added to foods and chewing gum as an artificial sweetener it's also found naturally in apples as well as stone fruits, including apricots, cherries, pears, and plums, although in very small amounts. It's also added to kids' cough syrup as well as other medicines and appears on the label as "420." Mannitol ("421") is another additive that will up your gas output. The problem is that because we lack the enzymes to break down a sugar alcohol like sorbitol our bacteria ferments them, causing not only gas but also serious bloating and even diarrhea.

Too much gas in the colon is what causes bloating—everybody's least favorite dinner party guest. Bloating occurs when we feel tight and full in the abdomen, which appears to swell up to the size of a second trimester pregnancy. Bloating isn't caused generally by swallowing excessive air but rather by the fermentation of waste, which produces gas. There *are* ways to control bloating, which generally involve controlling gas.

The many and varied possible causes of excessive gas

- not chewing food adequately

- eating too much

- swallowing air when eating too quickly

- lying down right after eating

- eating right before bedtime

- excessive consumption of alcohol or caffeine

- inadequate stomach acid

- too much stomach acid

- food intolerance and sensitivity

- antibiotics

- lack of healthy intestinal flora

- irritable bowel syndrome (IBS)

- colitis

- gallstones and gall bladder dysfunction

- candida-related complex

- stress

- anesthetics

- parasites

- pelvic organ dysfunction
- pancreatic dysfunction
- bleeding ulcers
- partial bowel obstruction
- constipation

If you want to minimize your gas output, look at the causes and see what you can eliminate from your life. Otherwise, there are always a few short-term solutions, including charcoal tablets that absorb gas, digestive enzymes (if inadequate stomach acid or lactose intolerance is your problem), herbal teas like ginger and peppermint, and over-the-counter antacids that break up gas bubbles in your upper GIT. These make it easier to burp and reduce bloating and farting. To achieve the same end, a lot of people (like Bill Clinton) swear by aloe vera juice.

A healthy dose of probiotics like acidophilus and bifidus (more on those wonder supplements later) will also help maintain a healthy balance of intestinal flora so that bacterial activity is working *for* you rather than *against* you. And don't forget, no matter what your loved ones tell you, it's better out than in.

Stools

Okay, here we get to the part that a lot of people really have a problem talking about. Or even *reading* about! But don't chicken out—you may learn something incredibly important to your health. And we promise not to be too gross.

On average, we eliminate between 100 and 150 grams of fecal matter every day. But what is it? Our stools are composed of around 75 percent water as well as bowel bacteria, undigested food and fiber, and intestinal cells. The interesting thing is that you can tell a huge amount about people from their stools. Most important, you can tell how well their digestive system is working.

A person with a healthy digestive system has stools that are big, round, softish, and not horrible smelling. Sure, they're not going to smell like roses, but a really noxious smell can mean that you've eaten something that disagrees with you, or you may even be sick. When we say stools should be big we mean not thin and snakey or ribbon-like. If they're the latter, your bowel is straining too much to move things forward and is perhaps not relaxed enough, especially at the exit point.

There is major disagreement among digestive healthcare practitioners about whether stools should float or sink. If your stools float, it could mean that there's too much gas or mucous in the stool. Mucous can indicate a number of problems. On the other hand, people who eat a lot of fiber and produce more gas than average often have floating poo as well. Much more important than whether it floats or sinks is whether or not it passes easily and regularly. So don't add the float versus sink issue to the list of things that can keep you awake in the middle of the night. Life is way too short.

Color-wise, stools should range from medium to dark brown. This is because of bilirubin, a waste product from worn-out red blood cells that's yellow in color. It's excreted in the bile and modified by colonic bacteria that make feces brown. If your stools are chronically pale brown or yellowish, you may be producing too little in the way of bile salts. If your stools are grayish white or very pale yellow for more than a few days, see your doctor, as this could indicate problems involving the liver, pancreas, or gall bladder, particularly gallstones blocking the bile duct. If your stools are black, you could be bleeding from somewhere along the GIT, so you should see your doctor. But be aware that iron supplements and too much licorice can darken your output as well.

The amount of water you drink and the way your body handles it will also determine the condition of your stools. We absorb a lot of water from waste in the bowel, and if we take in too little water there won't be enough left after absorption to keep the stool soft. Instead it will become hard and difficult to move, and can lead to constipation and hemorrhoids. This is one of the main reasons for having a diet high in fiber—fiber retains water so it keeps your stools big and soft.

But remember to drink extra water the more fiber you take in, or you can get very clogged up. Water will continue to be absorbed from fecal matter while it's in the colon so you really need to keep it moving. Otherwise, this alone can cause the stools to become compact and hard to pass.

On the other hand, when you have diarrhea your bowel is irritated so it's not absorbing *any* water, which is why the stools are runny and unformed. Because there's no time for the waste to be further broken down by bacteria, that's also why diarrhea is greenish and *really* hard on the nose. But the question on everyone's mind is, how *often* should I have a movement? Well, everyone's different, but there's no question that it's generally good to have *at least* one bowel movement a day. Any less than that and waste may get backed up and cause trouble. Even people who are fasting have some bowel movements, made of water, bacteria, and intestinal cells. Many people with very high-fiber diets and everything else in working order go three times a day! The important thing to understand is that there are individual variations. Some people only go three or four times a week and are perfectly healthy. The most significant indicators are whether you pass your stools *easily* and *regularly*. If you're not going regularly there are a lot of things you can do that you can read about in our exciting section on constipation, coming up shortly.

Urine

While peeing is not part of digestive function, it's a good indicator of your hydration levels, so you can't go wrong having a look at your pee every now and then.

Urine is the combination of waste molecules and water collected from the blood by the kidneys, and the system works best when there's enough water to dilute the waste. And if there's enough water to dilute and carry away the waste, there's probably enough to help you break down your food and maintain active, healthy bowels. Enough water means that your pee should be clear to pale yellow. If it's dark yellow or brownish, this is a sign that you're dehydrated to a point that can affect many of your body's functions, from waste clearance to digestion. If you take vitamin B supplements, they will color your pee a bright yellow and then fade through the day.

Blood in the urine can be a serious disease indicator, and should send you off to the doctor pronto.

Frequency of urination depends on a wide variety of factors, from the size of your bladder, to the outside air temperature, to the amount of exercise you do, to whether or not you're pregnant and of course how much water or fluid you ingest. In other words, there is no right number of times a day you should pee. The quality of your pee (how pale it is) is much more important than the quantity.

The Aztecs used to drink their urine to treat gastroin-

testinal disorders, but this application has yet to be scientifi-
cally tested. In any case, unless you have a urinary tract infection, most urine is sterile, so you won't be doing any serious
damage if you have a swig and see for yourself!

Two
Digestive Disorders

*B*ecause the digestive system is so complex and relies on so many organs and tissues outside the digestive tract, there are literally hundreds of things that can go wrong with it. Nearly all of us will experience at least one of many digestive disorders in our lifetimes, whether it's something as common as indigestion or as serious as colorectal cancer. The good news is that more and more research is revealing ways to combat and prevent these conditions, and in some cases the trick is a slight change in your diet and a few brisk walks every week. But for now, let's briefly review the variety of disorders and diseases that can affect your digestive system, and therefore your whole life.

Halitosis (bad breath)

Many people are still under the mistaken impression that all bad breath comes from unclean teeth, bacteria in the mouth, or gum disease. Hence the popularity of mouthwashes, mints, and toothpastes enhanced to "kill germs that can cause bad breath" or simply mask bad breath with the heavy scent of peppermint. Flossing will often eliminate odors that come from the mouth so try this first.

But while unclean teeth and the presence of bacteria can indeed cause bad breath, there are many other common causes that often originate in the gastrointestinal tract. The problem may be a digestive system that isn't working well or something in your bloodstream that's being released through your lungs (like alcohol or garlic). In some cases your digestive system may have been compromised by illness, and in others a restrictive diet might be the culprit. Anyone who knows someone who has been on the Atkins diet for a while can tell you that while weight loss is one of the triumphs of the regimen, sweet-smelling breath is not.

The point is that if you suffer from bad breath and you've tried every mouthwash, toothpaste, and breath freshener on the market, you might try looking a little lower down for the solution to your problem. Basically, a diet high in fiber, fresh fruit, vegetables, and properly cooked fish and meat will help. Lots of saturated fats will not help. But there may also be some underlying cause. Sometimes food intolerance or sensitivity can challenge the digestive system in such a way as to yield less than fragrant odors at your top end. A visit to either a medical doctor or a complementary therapist can help put you on the right track. There are some cities that even have halitosis clinics, so there are a lot of alternatives out there. Just don't give up and spend your life—and your money—gargling without results. And please don't just live with it. You may think no one else notices, but they're probably just being polite.

Important Note

No matter what your disorder, see your healthcare practitioner if you have trouble that isn't going away or if you have extreme symptoms. You can waste thousands of dollars on unnecessary or inadequate self-treatment, not to mention the time you spend feeling ill, missing out on work, family, friends, cocktail parties, etc. Or, your condition could worsen and even become irreversible. Whatever you do, don't just learn to live with pain or discomfort.

Indigestion and heartburn (reflux)

Indigestion, also called dyspepsia, is an umbrella term used to describe any mild pain, discomfort, or gas that result when our food doesn't sit well in our stomachs. Heartburn, also known as reflux, is one of the most common forms of indigestion, which feels like a burning pain in the middle of the chest. You may also feel a dull ache in the upper abdomen, nausea, or burp a lot. The causes are many (see opposite), so if you have persistent symptoms it's important to isolate the problem and fix it.

During pregnancy, heartburn can occur because the stomach is pushed up against the esophagus. Also, the muscles are more relaxed due to the hormone relaxin, which also makes the esophageal sphincter relax. Some causes of indigestion will affect certain people and not others, and most of the time the explanation for your indigestion is obvious and isn't life-threatening. Generally the solutions lie in simple food elimination or lifestyle changes. It usually doesn't take a specialist to work this out. For example, if you start burping only when you eat cheeseburgers and fries, they probably have something to do with it.

Other factors can be less obvious. A common condition that is often misdiagnosed is inadequate stomach acid, which many people mistake for *too much* acidity. If you have low levels of hydrochloric acid, you can't break down protein and are less able to kill bacteria and viruses that can then inhabit the bowel. Symptoms include burping as soon as you start eating, bloating, food sensitivities or allergies, dry lips, and feeling full after eating a small amount. You may be helped by taking digestive aid tablets, which are available in pharmacies and health food store. These can sometimes eliminate symptoms that have been plaguing you for years. But like all medications and supplements, you shouldn't take them indefinitely, and not without the advice of a professional.

The many and varied possible causes of indigestion

- overeating

- eating too fast

- eating right before you go to bed

- lying down or bending over after eating

- too much or too little stomach acid

- alcohol

- caffeine

- smoking

continued

- stress

- refined carbohydrates

- sugar

- chocolate (sad but true)

- fatty or oily foods

- hot and spicy foods

- foods like onions, garlic, tomatoes, or oranges

- cola drinks, carbonated drinks

- drinking too much fluid when you eat

- drugs (e.g., birth control pills, nitroglycerine, magnesium, NSAIDs—non-steroidal anti-inflammatory drugs such as aspirin)

- gallstones

- ulcers

- irritable bowel syndrome (IBS)

- food intolerances

- lack of exercise

- lack of fiber

- obesity

- heart disease

- stomach cancer

- pregnancy

While you may be helped by over-the-counter antacids, if the source of your trouble is in your diet then it's probably better to just drop the offending foods from your menu. Also, overconsumption of antacids can make your body actually produce *more* acid on its own and you've started a vicious cycle. You can also get "prokinetic" drugs by prescription that affect the way your stomach empties itself, basically by relieving tension in the stomach muscles. But there are possible side effects like cramps, muscle spasms, and diarrhea, so watch out.

Reflux occurs when stomach acid leaks back up into the esophagus because the valve has opened at the wrong moment, which also gives rise to a burning sensation. This can often occur when we lie down. The problem might be that the sphincter muscle is too relaxed (often caused by heavy drinking), or you could have a hiatus hernia, which occurs when the esophagus pushes through the diaphragm muscle. This often occurs in people who are overweight or have bad posture and the stomach has actually been pushed upward, compacting the esophagus. Postural correction or weight loss can help this, as can a treatment with manipulation by a trained visceral osteopath or chiropractor.

Most of the time reflux doesn't damage the esophagus, but sometimes it can cause inflammation called esophagitis, common among smokers. This can lead to scarring and narrowing of the esophagus, which requires treatment in the hospital. Or, the esophagus may gradually develop a mucous lining like the stomach. This is called Barrett's esophagus and can eventually lead to esophageal cancer.

Reflux, or heartburn, can be caused by the same things that cause other forms of indigestion, so you need to isolate the cause or causes in your particular case and then eliminate them.

If your indigestion is accompanied by any of the following symptoms, see your doctor right away:

- weight loss
- loss of appetite
- constant nausea
- difficulty swallowing
- vomiting blood or brown gritty matter
- dark blood in your stools.

If you have indigestion when you've never had it before and you're over forty, you should visit the doctor too. Or if you have what feels like heartburn or pain in the chest when you exert yourself that goes away when you rest, it may not be heartburn at all but angina, so get to the doctor, pronto.

Nausea and vomiting

While nausea and vomiting are not diseases, they are symptoms so common as to warrant their own section. While hard to define, nausea is the sensation of queasiness and discomfort in the stomach that is often accompanied by an urge to throw up. Vomiting, or throwing up, is the forced or unforced emptying of the stomach through the esophagus and mouth, also known as reverse peristalsis. Not a day at the beach.

There are many possible causes of nausea and vomiting, such as:

- food poisoning
- viral infection
- motion sickness
- pregnancy
- concussion, brain tumor, or other brain disorder
- overeating
- excessive alcohol intake

- migraine headache
- appendicitis
- blocked intestine
- drugs (both prescription and recreational)
- food intolerance
- liver disease
- kidney disease
- heart attack
- nervous system disorder
- some forms of cancer
- severe pain
- exposure to chemical toxins
- high fever
- whooping cough or other chronic cough
- stomach ulcer
- bulimia
- profound disgust

The cause of your nausea or vomiting may be obvious, such as pregnancy, when many women experience "morning sickness," especially in the first trimester. Also known as morning-noon-and-night sickness to many, this condition can best be treated by drinking peppermint, ginger, or licorice teas, eating small, frequent meals, and generally trying to distract yourself with things like fixing up the nursery and watching your favorite DVDs. Unfortunately, there is no cure.

Motion sickness is incredibly common, especially on long car trips in the heat with small children who just had the cheeseburger, fries, and shake at the last pit stop. The associated nausea and vomiting can largely be prevented by over-the-counter tablets that should be administered before the trip. Many a start to summer vacation has been saved by this simple but crucial step.

A lot of cancer patients undergoing chemotherapy find that their nausea can be suppressed through the use of marijuana, but while the clinical effect is accepted, its legal use is not. So that choice is up to you.

Other causes of nausea and vomiting may be less obvious, and if your symptoms persist for more than a couple of days, or you are unable to keep food down at all, see your doctor. But go to your doctor *immediately* if nausea or vomiting are also accompanied by rapid breathing or pulse, high fever, blood in the vomit that looks like coffee grounds, major headache or stiff neck, lethargy, mental vagueness, or acute pain in the abdomen.

Self-induced vomiting, or bulimia, is a condition that will have dreadful long-term effects on everything from your gastrointestinal tract to your teeth, your breath, and certainly your self-esteem, so you need to get counseling as soon as you can.

No matter what the cause of your vomiting, you need to replace fluids and electrolytes, especially if you've been hurling for a while. Stick to clear fluids like water, sports drinks, broths, and teas, as well as other electrolyte solutions available from drugstores, and try drinking small amounts frequently to begin with. And just say no to that sixth beer.

Gastroenteritis

Gastroenteritis is the irritation and inflammation of the digestive tract leading to abdominal pain, vomiting, and diarrhea—the passing of unformed, watery stools. With a typical case, you may also experience weakness, fever or chills, and dehydration. Gastroenteritis has a wide variety of causes, including:

- food or water poisoning (from viruses, bacteria, and parasites)
- food allergies
- food intolerances
- alcohol abuse
- smoking
- bad diet
- vitamin and mineral deficiencies
- vitamin and mineral overdoses
- laxative abuse

• radiation or chemotherapy
• drugs (including antibiotics).

Let's look at some of the causes of food poisoning in particular more closely.

Food poisoning

There are different kinds of food poisoning, some of which trigger symptoms within an hour of eating contaminated food and others that may take from a day or so to months or even years to make themselves known. With the first type there will usually be no more than a day or two of cramps and diarrhea. Bacteria are usually the culprits, but poisoning can also be caused by molds, yeasts, and viruses.

Most cases of food poisoning in the United States are caused by bacteria. One of these is salmonella, which can lurk in raw or undercooked meats, especially chicken. But believe it or not, it can also be present in chocolate, dried coconut, eggs, and peanut butter. Leaving uncooked meat near other foods (even in the fridge!) can lead to cross-contamination, so be very careful when wrapping and storing meats.

The other common bacteria causing food poisoning is *Escherichia coli O157:H7* or E. coli for short. There are hundreds of strains of E. coli, but the one with the numbers after it is the one that can make us sick. It comes from the intestines of healthy cattle, and can get mixed into beef when it's ground for our consumption. Sufficiently high temperatures will kill it. That's why it's vital to cook ground beef thoroughly—the days of enjoying your burger pink in the middle are over. The bacteria are also found on cows' udders so it can be present in raw (unpasteurized) milk, which is best avoided for this reason. E. coli can also be spread by infected stools, typically from toddlers whose handwashing habits aren't perfect, and from sewage-contaminated water.

The nasty strain of E. coli often causes severe bloody diarrhea and abdominal cramps, which usually subside in from five to ten days without any treatment except fluids and electrolytes. Antibiotics and anti-diarrhea drugs can often makes things worse. In some people, usually kids under the age of five or the elderly, the infection can lead to a complication called hemolytic uremic syndrome, which involves the destruction of red blood cells and eventually kidney failure. This condition accounts for the small number of deaths every year associated with E. coli, and it's one more reason to order your burger well done or opt for the pasta and salad.

Other bacteria can thrive in cooked food that sits in the fridge for more than two or three days, so don't keep leftovers for longer! Bacteria can be killed only by *thorough* re-heating, so take care especially when microwaving, which can give uneven results. And then there are the bacteria that can spread to food when we sneeze or let infected cuts or sores come into contact with food.

Parasites are microorganisms that live off other organisms (like us!) and can cause food poisoning where symptoms may emerge right away or maybe not for a long time. Two of the most common varieties are giardia and cryptosporidium, and can come from untreated water, unwashed food, unwashed hands, raw meat and fish, and pets. Our stomach acid can kill parasites like giardia—that's its function—but it doesn't work 100 percent of the time. If you're unlucky enough to play host to a parasite, you're likely to have the usual symptoms of gastroenteritis plus a fever. Parasites can also damage your digestive enzymes like lactase, which you need for digesting milk sugar, so, if you're affected, avoid milk products for a few days or they could make your symptoms worse. And that's only in the short term. If you have long-term intestinal parasites, you may have digestive problems stemming from an imbalance of your intestinal flora but also symptoms of arthritis, chronic fatigue, and even mental and emotional problems. The trouble with parasites is that they're not always easy to detect, and may not show up in a stool sample test.

One of the least appealing types of parasites has to be the worm, which can live in your gut and comes in varieties as small as an inch, and as long as twenty-six feet (no kidding). Worms can cause diarrhea, constipation, an itchy anus, and weight loss through malabsorption of nutrients. Depending on the type of worm, treatment can be easy or it can take months. Definitely see your doctor if worms are suspected. And if they're confirmed, treat your whole family at the same time as yourself.

One might think that because we're more aware of hygiene and other factors in food management we're suffering with parasites less than we used to. Well, think again. Parasitic invasions are becoming more and more prevalent because we eat out more, get more take-out, have more kids at day care and pre-school, travel more, and consume food from a wider variety of sources than ever. In other words, by not preparing our own food we're taking a risk. But you've got to have a life, right? There are a lot of simple things you can do to keep from falling prey to parasites and other microorganisms, at least in your own home. So just be aware of what you can do to prevent poisoning and what you should do if you fail.

How to prevent food poisoning at home

- Wash your hands thoroughly after using the bathroom, doing the gardening, and handling animals, including house pets.

- Don't sleep with your pets.

- Regularly de-worm your pets.

- When shopping, buy food last (especially meat, fish, and dairy) that needs to be refrigerated, and don't let it sit in a hot car while you stop for a coffee.

- Keep your fridge temperature set below 26 degrees Fahrenheit.

- Thaw frozen food in the fridge. It will take longer but it's safer than leaving it out or letting it sit in water.

- Wash your hands thoroughly before and after food preparation, and rinse them even between preparing different foods.

- Wash fruit and vegetables thoroughly.

- Keep countertops and cutting boards clean, and don't set meats, especially poultry, on wooden surfaces.

- Keep utensils clean and wash between use on different foods.

continued

- Replace sponges frequently and use clean dish towels.

- Cook foods to over 212 degrees Fahrenheit and reheat left-overs so they're hot, not just warm.

- After you cook, don't let leftovers sit around but put them straight into the fridge (but not in hot containers!).

- Keep cooked and uncooked foods separate, and wrap them thoroughly.

- Maintain healthy levels of friendly flora in your gut by taking probiotics if you need to (more on them later!).

When you're abroad, especially in countries where the hygiene is questionable, drink bottled or filtered water and consider taking digestive aid tablets to bolster the potency of your own stomach acid. You can also get tablets to add to water to neu-tralize dangerous invaders. It's also best to avoid salads and other uncooked foods, unless you want to spend half your vacation on the toilet.

How to treat food poisoning

Vomiting and diarrhea cause you to lose lots of fluids, as well as vitamins and minerals that have to be replaced. So the first thing you need to do is drink water and clear fluids like herbal teas and broths, but *also* special products available from the pharmacist that come in powder form in premeasured packets that will replace your electrolytes. You simply mix them with water and will feel better very quickly after drinking the solution. This will replace electrolytes that are essential salts, including sodium, potassium, calcium, magnesium, and others that become quickly depleted with diarrhea. Some sports drinks can also help here.

Teas that are especially kind to the belly are chamomile, slippery elm, ginger, and raspberry. Slippery elm powder in water can also work wonders.

In many cases it's best to avoid dairy products, as it will take a few days for your milk sugar digesting enzymes to reappear, although many people actually find them easy to take, and dairy can be a good way to replace your electrolytes.

It's also smart to replace the friendly intestinal flora you've unloaded along with all the bad stuff your body rightly rejected. At any health food store you can buy a variety of probiotics, but get advice from the naturopath or your practitioner about types and dosages.

Important Note

All infants with symptoms of gastroenteritis should be taken to a doctor or the emergency room of your hospital. Life-threatening dehydration in babies can occur very quickly, so you don't want to mess around. This means that if your little one has had diarrhea for longer than a couple of hours, is crying, has dry mouth, or the fontanel (soft spot in skull) appears sunken, get moving.

Forget about solid food for a day or two, and when you do start eating again, begin with bland foods like rice and bread. Then slowly graduate to steamed vegetables and keep proteins for last. Hold off as long as possible on raw foods, fatty foods, refined sugars, alcohol, and caffeine. And don't take aspirin or ibuprofen, as they can further irritate your GIT.

There are medications you can take to *stop* vomiting and diarrhea, but these should only be taken under a doctor's supervision. When you have gastroenteritis, your body reacts the way it does because it's trying to get rid of something that's bad for you. So whether you like it or not, it's usually best to go with the flow, unless it's gone on too long.

If your symptoms persist for more than two days, and you're not responding to treatment, go to the doctor. You should also see your practitioner if you see dark blood or mucous in your stools, if you have a high fever, bad abdominal or rectal pain, or if you have an unquenchable thirst or haven't urinated in six hours.

It's really important to watch children of *any* age with gastroenteritis. They will usually need a practitioner's attention, and you'll benefit from advice about fluids and a restrictive diet for a while.

Another thing to be aware of is that a great deal of childhood diarrhea is caused by the consumption of too much fruit juice. A lot of parents are under the mistaken impression that a lot of fruit juice is a healthy alternative to soft drinks, but it can actually give them a chronic case of the runs. So limit their fruit juice intake, and always dilute their juice with water, one-to-one. Those colorful juice boxes may be convenient but they can be dangerous—like so many nice things—if used excessively. They're okay for school lunches, but when the kids are home, dilute their fruit juice and think about something as novel as milk with dinner.

Constipation

When the nutrients have been absorbed from your food and what's left passes into the colon it becomes waste, or what you'd recognize as fecal matter. It's important that this undigested matter visit the colon for a little while so that fermentation takes place, but you don't want it hanging around for too long. And all too often that's exactly what happens. Unfortunately, while it sits there more waste is channeled in behind it, until it becomes hard and compact. The longer it sits there the harder it is to expel because of compaction and also because water continues to be absorbed. This unfortunate and incredibly common condition is called constipation, and everyone who's ever had it knows how awful that sick-all-over feeling is.

The sick-all-over feeling is due to a combination of symptoms that include bloating, lethargy, and a sensation of heaviness.

The most common causes of constipation are:

- lack of water
- lack of fiber
- lack of exercise
- stress
- hormone swings
- travel
- certain foods (e.g. cheese, fried food)
- age
- certain medications.

Waste needs to be relatively soft to be pushed through the bowel, so you need to consume a lot of water—more than most people do. Eight to ten glasses a day will make a world of difference if you suffer from constipation and your water intake isn't that high. The minimum recommended dosage of water per day (eight glasses) is being called into question, and there's no doubt that many people don't need that much. But consuming more water very often helps people who suffer from constipation, and drinking eight glasses a day isn't going to hurt them unless there are unusual complicating factors.

If you suffer from constipation, one of the niftiest tricks is to drink two glasses of water as soon as you get up in the morning. This action seems to set your GIT's peristaltic waves in motion, and it has a domino effect.

The other easy fix is fiber. There will be a whole section devoted to the wonders of fiber later so suffice it for now to say that most people with chronic constipation don't get nearly enough fiber in their diets. In fact most people who never even get constipated don't consume enough fiber. Fiber doesn't actually get absorbed as a nutrient but it does absorb water, so when it travels into the bowel along with the rest of your waste it makes it softer and easier to move. Even without changing your diet in a major way you can introduce fiber by taking a teaspoon or two of psyllium husks—available at health food stores—mixed in a glass of water, and then following that with *another* glass of water. Be sure to drink the glass with the psyllium husks quickly, or the solution will be too thick to swallow comfortably. You will experience some bloating at first, but gradually this will subside as your bowel gets used to the new volume of bulk. There are also fiber products available at pharmacies, but they often have sweeteners and other additives that you don't necessarily want.

Drinking licorice tea is a delicious and easy way to keep mild constipation at bay, especially if you drink it daily.

Perhaps the best way to prevent constipation is to exercise regularly. *We cannot stress this enough!* Runners and power walkers rarely get constipated. People with chronic constipation are often those who sit all day at a desk or behind the wheel of a car or truck, and then all night in front of a TV and don't do anything to compensate for it. This lifestyle is murder on your bowel, which needs lots of movement, healthy circulation, and the help of good old gravity. So get off your butts and shake things up with some regular exercise and avoid that feeling of having waste stagnating and building up inside you. Even if you have a sedentary job and lifestyle, just half an hour four or five days a week of fairly vigorous exercise will keep you regular.

Working long shifts or just long hours can also throw your digestive cycle out of whack, as can eating at irregular times, skipping breakfast, or not going to the toilet when you feel the urge. If you can avoid any of these things, do, otherwise you might find yourself to be regularly irregular. One of the other major contributors to constipation is stress, because many people hold their anxiety in their gut rather than (or even as well as!) in their backs or necks or jaws like a lot of other people. So if that's your problem, you need to find a way to manage your stress. You can't eliminate stress entirely and you wouldn't want to. But you have to find a way to limit the way it can affect your body negatively. Whether it's with aromatherapy, meditation, yoga, basketball, or basket weaving, you'll have more regular movements if you can learn to control your stress levels. More on stress management later.

More women than men get constipated, and this is due to hormone swings. Hormone receptors line the entire GIT and there's an intimate, if sometimes troubled, relationship between hormone levels and bowel movements. Because of this, many women get constipated just before their periods and also during pregnancy because of the hormone relaxin, which relaxes the muscles of the GIT as well as pelvic muscles. Things also are not helped by the growing baby pressing against the bowel and compacting its contents. So whatever you do to prevent or cope with constipation in general, do more of it at these times.

Travel is the other bane of the constipated, and there are many theories as to why. Some suggest that the cabin pressure in airplanes forces the compacting of the bowel, but those who travel in cars and trains often experience the same problems. It's more likely that it has something to do with sitting for long periods in confined spaces, eating foods low in fiber and not drinking enough water. So when you travel bring some fruit to snack on rather than opting for the hot chips at the truck stop, and bring a bottle of water that you continually refill. It's also undoubtedly true that a lot of us are inhibited by the idea of having a bowel movement in strange toilets. Sometimes the atmosphere in the bathroom at the gas station isn't exactly conducive to a stress-free visit. There's nothing like relaxing in the comfort of the throne in your own bathroom, but you should try to find ways to transcend your alien surroundings if you don't want to get blocked up on the road.

With foods, it's usually pretty easy to figure out what blocks you up. For many it's anything that's made with lots of oil, like potato chips or fried foods, and cheese is a common bowel movement inhibitor. In general, fat slows the stomach emptying process and takes longer to digest, so a high-fat diet slows gut transit time and will contribute to constipation. If you suspect a certain food or a type of diet might be at the root of your problem, alter your eating habits for a week or so and see if your motions get more regular. If so, change your diet so that you limit the offending foods to the point where you become regular. When you *do* eat foods that tend to block you up, increase your fluid and fiber intake.

Sometimes, constipation can be relieved with massage, administered by a professional massage therapist, a sensitive friend, or even yourself! Simply lie on your back with cushions under your head and your knees so your belly muscles are relaxed, and then slowly, gently and deeply massage in the direction your bowel is supposed to move—up the right side, across the tummy and then down on the left. If you feel any pain or blockage, stop and try it *very gently*.

Magnesium can also prevent constipation, as it relieves and prevents muscular cramps and spasms that can contribute to a lack of motion. Never forget that your bowel is made of muscle and needs the same nutrients that all your muscles need. It's best to eat foods like green vegetables and cereals that are rich in magnesium rather than overdosing on supplements which are not recommended, not required, nor cheap. And don't forget the humble prune. Beloved by millions of constipation sufferers worldwide, good old prunes can get things moving when more costly and sophisticated treatments fail.

A very strong word of warning about laxatives. Most people who suffer with constipation have resorted to using laxatives, and they know that there's nothing more wonderful than that explosive relief when their bowels finally empty. But this is a quick fix that can be very dangerous, depending on what kind you use. There are two kinds—stimulant cathartics that are very aggressive, and bulking agents, stool softeners, and lubricants that bother the bowel far less. Stimulant cathartics irritate the intestinal lining, provoking the same kind of response that food poisoning does—cramps and diarrhea. In the process, the bowel's natural motion is inhibited and it seems to forget what its job is, because something else is doing the job instead. So the kind of motion that took one laxative tablet last week might take two or three this week. And four next week. And so on. Also, over time, the nerves to the colon become less sensitive. This sort of laxative abuse is very common and can eventually make your bowel pretty useless. So go with the other solutions like fluids and fiber and exercise next time you get that backed up feeling, and then keep them up so you aren't ever tempted to reach for the laxatives again.

Hemorrhoids

Not a pleasant subject, hemorrhoids are an awful pain in the butt that affects more people than would like to admit it. Hemorrhoids are actually varicose veins (abnormally dilated veins) in the tissue at the bottom of the anal canal that helps to keep your anus closed. They occur when this tissue gets over-filled with blood, often from straining or pushing when trying to have a bowel movement. Hemorrhoids are another reason you don't want to be constipated and have hard, dry stools. When you strain, your veins bulge, and they can easily tear and bleed. This isn't nice.

Hemorrhoids can be caused by the same things that cause constipation, but also by heavy lifting, obesity, pregnancy, and just plain unlucky genetics. To prevent them, do all the things that can prevent constipation, and if you need something topical to soothe the area, talk to the naturopath or go to your health food store. Pharmacists also have a variety of topical treatments, but nothing beats prevention!

Irritable bowel syndrome (IBS)

IBS affects somewhere between 15 percent and 20 percent of all adults in the United States. It's one of the most common reasons that people visit their GPs, with about half of all gastrointestinal complaints caused by IBS. It's three times more common among women than men, and it's on the increase. But what is it?

IBS isn't technically a disease, but a label for a group of symptoms. However, experts believe that interaction between the brain and the bowel is abnormal in people with IBS. The result is that the nerves in the gut and those controlling the gut are particularly sensitive. Foods, stress, gas, and other stimuli that would pose no problem to others can cause contractions in the gut resulting in discomfort, pain, and even diarrhea.

No matter what the cause, symptoms of IBS can include:

• constipation, usually alternating with diarrhea
• abdominal pain and cramping
• bloating
• flatulence
• thin or small stools
• mucous in stools
• headaches
• fatigue
• anxiety
• irritability.

Essentially, IBS occurs when peristalsis in the bowel is irregular. It seems to forget both when to move and when *not* to! Which can be very distressing. The tricky thing is that the causes of IBS can be rather elusive, but with a little detective work you can usually figure out what triggers an episode in your case.

Some of the common triggers for IBS include:

• stress
• lactose intolerance
• caffeine
• chocolate
• alcohol

- spicy foods
- carbonated drinks
- lack of fiber
- too much fiber
- female hormones.

A recent study suggested that a bacterium, *Mycobacterium avium paratuberculosis* (MAP), which is linked to Crohn's disease, may also be a factor in IBS. Certainly in laboratory animals MAP inflames the nerves of the gut, and may also do so in humans. Obviously more study into this connection needs to be done, especially if something as simple as a course of antibiotics could relieve IBS sufferers' symptoms.

If you have symptoms of IBS, especially ones that aren't going away after a few days, it's important to see your doctor to eliminate other causes and discuss a treatment plan. A GP can take a medical history, perform a physical examination, and order tests. These might include a stool sample to see if there's any bleeding, X-rays, or a colonoscopy (viewing the colon through a flexible tube inserted through the anus), which is performed by a gastroenterologist who can determine if you have a more serious disease.

The keys to treatment for IBS are diet and stress management, and your doctor may also give you laxatives or prescriptions for anti-spasmodics as well as drugs that actually slow down the movement of food through the bowel. These should just be taken in the short term, as drugs can actually worsen your condition over time and also have unwanted side effects. You may also get a prescription for tranquilizers or antidepressants if stress rather than food seems to bring on your irritable bowel.

To figure out what foods make your bowel unhappy, keep a journal for a few weeks describing what you eat and then how your bowel reacts within a day or two. It should be pretty obvious what foods are giving you trouble. Then, just eliminate those foods from your diet and see if you feel better after six to eight weeks. Then comes the exciting part: the food challenge. Eat one of the suspected trigger foods and see how you react after a day or two. Keep adding suspect foods at least a day after each other until you've confirmed what the culprits are. Then simply avoid the guilty foods to avoid further episodes of IBS.

There are also a lot of treatments available at pharmacies and health food stores, which you can obtain without a prescription, that might help alleviate symptoms, such as aloe vera (available in capsules or juice), slippery elm, and other herbs. Probiotics like acidophilus and bifidus will also help maintain a regular bowel.

Medical practitioners disagree about the connection between IBS and more serious diseases. Some believe there is no connection, while others suggest that IBS may lead to ulcerative colitis and even increase the risk of colorectal cancer. But either way, it's a good idea to eliminate the triggers for IBS that may also be related to other disorders.

Ulcers

In the old days the accepted wisdom was that stomach ulcers were caused by excess stomach acid induced by stress, but we now know the truth: most stomach ulcers (also known as peptic ulcers) are caused by a bacterium called *Helicobacter pylori* (Hp) that's passed down to infants through families. Certainly stress can make an ulcer worse, but the bacterium is the root of the problem. Around 30 percent of us have *Helicobacter pylori* living in the mucous lining of our stomachs, but most of us don't have any symptoms. Of the 30 percent infected, around 10 percent of those will develop an ulcer in the stomach or duodenum.

Another commonly held myth is that an ulcer is a hole. It's actually a small, sore indentation that occurs when that area of the stomach lining loses its top layers.

Symptoms of ulcers include either intermittent or per-sistent indigestion, pain in the upper middle of your abdomen, burning either any time or when you eat, and nausea, especially after eating. There are several ways to test for the presence of *Helicobacter pylori*: a breath test, a blood test, or a biopsy acquired through an endoscopy (flexible tube inserted through the mouth and esophagus to the stomach).

The great news is that *Helicobacter pylori* bacteria are usually wiped out after taking a couple of kinds of antibiotics and acid suppressants for a week or two. However, it's a good idea to be retested afterwards because a small percentage of sufferers need another course of drugs to really knock out the bacteria.

But bacteria are not the only cause of stomach ulcers. Ulcers can be created by excessive exposure to common, over-the-counter non-steroidal anti-inflammatory drugs (NSAIDs) including aspirin and ibuprofen among others. This is very common among arthritis sufferers or people with chronic pain who take these drugs for long periods of time. New NSAIDs have been developed that still do the job but don't affect the stomach, so ask your doctor or pharmacist about them if you have stomach trouble.

Ulcers can also be caused by abuse of steroids such as cortisone, as well as too much alcohol (especially on an empty stomach!), and/or cigarette consumption. Once again, a consistently unhealthy lifestyle will get you into trouble.

In more uncommon cases, ulcers can be brought on by Crohn's disease (more on that later) or Zollinger-Ellison syndrome, where a hormonal imbalance can trigger the production of too much stomach acid. Cancer, or lymphoma of the stomach, may also cause ulcers, although the relationship between them is controversial and unclear.

Peptic ulcers are usually not that serious, but if untreated they *can* lead to things you'd much rather avoid, including bleeding. If an ulcer penetrates to an artery in the wall of the stomach or duodenum you could vomit blood that looks something like coffee grounds after interacting with stomach acid, or you could pass blood in your bowel movements that will look very dark to black. If either occurs, go straight to your doctor.

An untreated ulcer could also, in rare cases, go right through the intestinal wall, letting acid leak into the abdominal cavity causing peritonitis, which is a very painful infection demanding emergency surgery.

Another uncommon ulcer complication is pyloric stenosis, which occurs when there is an ulcer at the junction between the stomach and the duodenum that forms a scar restricting the pylorus—the valve at the bottom of the stomach. Symptoms include frequent vomiting and feeling full, and the condition may require surgery.

In the old days, surgery called a vagotomy was often performed to reduce the secretion of acid by the stomach glands. This is rarely done today, as medication and lifestyle changes usually do the trick.

Food allergies, intolerance, and sensitivity

There is a huge amount of confusion about food allergies, intolerance, and sensitivity, not only among the public, but in the press and even in the various healthcare professions themselves. Part of this is due to the way words are misused, and part of it is due to outright disagreement. In some cases, anecdotal evidence piles up but clinical studies fail to be done. In other cases, studies are carried out but their methods, results, and conclusions are questioned. There is bound to be a lot of controversy surrounding the subject for a long time, so what follows is an attempt to present a basic overview of the issues.

The first important thing to understand is the differences between an allergy and intolerance, and intolerance and sensitivity. Confusion abounds when these terms are used interchangeably, as they so often are.

Food allergy

This occurs when a food stimulates the immune system to react, usually fairly quickly (often in minutes), although in some cases, within hours or even days. Although this sort of food allergy is fairly rare, foods that commonly trigger an immune response are peanuts and shellfish. In extreme cases, the sufferer can go into anaphylactic shock, which involves swelling of the face and mouth and increasingly severe breathing difficulty. If the sufferer doesn't already have his or her own emergency kit (which contains injectable adrenaline) this reaction demands a fast trip to the hospital, and can result in death if left untreated. Sometimes the sufferer doesn't even have to eat the offending food but can absorb it through the skin (like peanut butter on another child's hand) or even inhale it through the air (like peanut protein in the air on a plane) and have an acute allergic reaction. These sorts of allergies need to be taken very seriously.

If a food allergy is suspected, your GP can refer you to an allergist for either skin or blood tests. Skin tests are the most common, in which the allergist pricks or scrapes the skin with extracts of a variety of foods and other allergens. After twenty minutes or so, something like a mosquito bite will appear if there is an allergic reaction to any of the tested substances. Sometimes you may be allergic but not react to the test, and will have to find other ways to determine the cause of your troubles.

Food intolerance

This occurs when there is a congenital (existing from birth) inability to digest a particular food, and has nothing to do with the immune system. For example, milk intolerance is the inability to digest lactose, which is the sugar in milk. The reason for this is that the sufferer lacks the digestive enzyme lactase, required to break down milk sugar. So, if someone who is lactose intolerant drinks milk, undigested lactose goes to the bowel where bacteria ferment it, causing diarrhea, gas, and other symptoms of IBS.

Food intolerance is much more common than food allergies and can affect entire races of people, the way lactose intolerance affects high percentages of African American, Australian Aboriginal, African, Asian, and Mediterranean people. More women than men are lactose intolerant, suggesting that there is also a hormonal link.

The trick to living with lactose intolerance is simply to eliminate excessive amounts of lactose from your diet, or to use enzyme tablets or drops that you can add to milk that help break down the lactose. Dairy milk, ice cream, and some yogurt have lactose, but—and this is a nice thing to hear—butter, cream, and cheese have almost none. Usually, a small amount of lactose isn't a problem for the intolerant, so you can have milk in your tea or coffee without making yourself sick. There is some evidence that people with lactose intolerance can more easily digest raw (unpasteurized) milk, but it can be somewhat difficult to find, as not many stores carry it. In any case, it's up to you to discover your tolerance levels.

Lactose intolerance can be diagnosed with a breath test, but usually it's easy to tell whether you have it from your own food experiences. Another common food intolerance is known as celiac disease, which is the inability to digest gluten, a protein found in grains including wheat, rye, barley, and oats. Unlike lactose intolerance, there is no missing enzyme or component that causes the intolerance. We do know that there is a clear genetic link.

What happens in sufferers is that the undigested gluten gradually wears down the intestinal lining so that sufferers are unable to absorb nutrients in their food, potentially leading to malnutrition or worse. This can also lead to leaky gut syndrome, where molecules normally too large to be absorbed can penetrate the bowel wall causing further problems. When tested, some people turn out to have celiac disease but have no symptoms, while others can have extreme symptoms. Others still can tolerate gluten only moderately well.

Like other food intolerance, the symptoms of celiac disease are the same as those with IBS—bloating, constipation and diarrhea, flatulence, abdominal pain, and mucous in the stools.

Unfortunately, there is no cure for celiac disease, and

people with symptoms need to avoid gluten for good. Also unfortunately for them, wheat has the most gluten of all the grains and is the most commonly used grain in our society, present in most breads, cereals, and pasta. The good news is that corn and rice are gluten-free, so if you suffer, start dusting off those recipes for risotto. And of course you can also get gluten-free breads and pastas at your local health food store, and although they may take some time to get used to, you could also be surprised at how tasty they are. Celiac disease can be accurately (in 95 percent of cases) diagnosed with a blood test, although an endoscopy is the surefire way to tell.

Intolerance to many other foods is common, including everything from chocolate to wheat (which is not the same as celiac disease). Ultimately it's up to you to figure out which food or foods you can't tolerate, and eliminate them from your diet. But be very careful not to deprive yourself of vital nutrients in the meantime. If you have a food intolerance you should consult a nutritional expert to help you design a diet that provides you with everything you need to stay healthy. Many people avoid foods unnecessarily and deprive themselves of essential nutrients.

Food sensitivity

This is different from an allergy or intolerance because it doesn't involve the immune system, and it's something that may only be temporary, not something you're born with and must live with for the rest of your life. Food sensitivity is incredibly common, and is often a postrecovery by-product of another disease. For example, in the short term, after you've had a bout of food poisoning you can't digest milk because a parasite has rendered your lactase inert. But this doesn't mean that you're lactose intolerant. It just means that you have a temporary sensitivity to lactose because of the gastroenteritis.

Another example of temporary food sensitivity is when you may have had glandular fever that resulted in postviral syndrome—a condition whereby your delayed recovery from the virus has led to sensitivities to everything from wheat to preservatives and flavorings in food such as MSG. But this doesn't mean that you're going to be intolerant of these foods forever. It *does* mean that you need to rebuild your digestive system and recover from the virus before you can start pigging out again on BLT sandwiches and Chinese take-out.

Food sensitivities can also be triggered by overexposure to the same food. What many people perceive as an "allergy" to wheat may simply be a sensitivity that developed because they simply consume too much of it. Wheaties for breakfast, a muffin for morning snack, a sandwich on wheat bread for lunch, and pasta for dinner may sound healthy, but a diet like that is an easy way to develop a negative reaction.

Some have theorized that we have an especially difficult time with grains because human beings have only been consuming them in any quantity for the past 12,000 years and our digestive systems haven't sufficiently evolved to cope. It's certainly true that the rise in obesity is partly due to the over-consumption of refined grains in bread, pasta, pizza, cookies, croissants, pies, cakes, muffins, and breakfast cereal. But the reasons for refined grain sensitivity are not totally clear. Equally, there is much research that demonstrates the benefits of *whole* grains. So the solution is to cut back on refined grains and bulk up on whole-grain breads and cereals.

Confusing food sensitivities with allergies and intolerance is one of the most common mistakes people make these days, with everyone terrified that they're "allergic" to wheat or garlic or milk or even tap water. It hasn't helped that the press jumps on every new story about the potential dangers lurking in our foods, and beats it up until there's a completely unjustified climate of fear about everything we put in our mouths.

The fact is that food sensitivities are incredibly common, but eliminating the offending food for some time (anywhere from a couple of days to a couple of months, depending on the case) and then reintroducing it can generally reverse them. If you get a bad reaction, then go off the food for longer. Otherwise, you may be fine, but do consider not having something like wheat five times a day if that's what made you feel ill in the first place. Of course there's a chance that you may stay sensitive to a food forever. Many people who could happily consume family-size blocks of chocolate when they were young become wildly dyspeptic if they indulge in a couple of M&Ms as adults. So you may have to give up chocolate for life. Either that or put up with some occasional dyspepsia.

The symptoms of food sensitivity are the same as those for food intolerance, but the severity can be of varying degrees. Not only are the usual digestive discomforts blamed on food sensitivities, but fatigue, fluid retention, headaches, stuffy noses, skin disorders, vagueness, anxiety, and depression are also said by many experts to be caused by our inability to process certain foods.

The idea of the connection between asthma and food allergies, intolerance, or sensitivity is very controversial, and while many practitioners believe that difficulties digesting certain foods can trigger asthma, most of the medical establishment blames allergens like dust mites or animal hair for asthmatic reactions rather than foods.

It is true that food sensitivities seem to be on the rise, and there are several theories as to why. It may have something to do with the fact that we eat a far greater variety of foods than in the past. Many doctors, nutritionists, and naturopaths also believe that the typical diet in developed countries like the United States and Australia eventually wears down the intestinal tract. With grotesque amounts of additives, preservatives, saturated fats, sugars, and flavorings in our foods, as well as the overconsumption of refined carbohydrates and caffeine, it seems inevitable that the digestive system will suffer. This fact underlines the need to return to healthier eating if we don't want to spend the rest of our lives feeling sick.

While the elimination of offending foods will help you avoid symptoms of food allergies, intolerance, and sensitivity, there are many things you can do to help stave off short-term indigestion, especially in the case of mild sensitivities. It can help to take some herbal bitters in water a little while before a meal, or even just a little lemon squeezed in water. Digestive aid tablets, available at pharmacies and health food stores, can also help, but should not be taken all the time or for extended periods. As with any ongoing condition, you should consult a practitioner to figure out a treatment plan and learn to distinguish between allergies, intolerance, and sensitivity, as the treatment for each is very different.

Inflammatory bowel disease (colitis and Crohn's disease)

Inflammatory bowel disease (IBD) is a collective term that includes *colitis*, *ulcerative colitis*, and *Crohn's disease*, and like so many other digestive disorders all varieties are on the increase in Western societies. The picture should be getting clearer and clearer that digestive health depends on diet!

Colitis is inflammation of the bowel, while ulcerative colitis occurs when the inflammation has led to ulceration. Crohn's disease is inflammation anywhere on the intestinal tract, usually in the ileum (the last part of the small intestine). The inflammation can go through all layers of the intestinal lining, possibly into the nearby lymph nodes. The symptoms for all IBDs are abdominal pain and diarrhea, and with ulcerative colitis and Crohn's disease there can also be blood and mucous in the stools, weight loss, fatigue, deficiencies including anemia, as well as skin disorders. With Crohn's disease the pain is often concentrated in the lower right abdomen.

IBD may be related to an immune dysfunction, where the body attacks its own tissue, but most recent studies also confirm that there is a clear dietary link. People who suffer from IBD generally have a diet much higher in refined carbohydrates, sugars, and saturated fats (think junk food!) and lower in fiber than non-sufferers, although this isn't always true. This explains why Crohn's disease and ulcerative colitis have significantly increased in countries with a "Western" diet (the U.S., Europe, and Australia) in the last two decades. There may also be a viral connection, on top of a genetic predisposition.

And if you think the problem may have something to do with racial chemistry or body types, think again. The rate of digestive diseases including IBD used to be comparatively low in Japan, but as the Japanese have adopted a Western diet so their rates of IBD have increased. Another example of the "civilizing" effect of Western culture.

A recent study in Britain also discovered a link between Crohn's disease and a bacterium found in some milk called *Mycobacterium avium paratuberculosis* (MAP). The bacteria were present in about 2 percent of pasteurized milk in Britain, and figures may be similar in the United States.

This finding suggests that treatment with antibiotics specifically designed to fight the bacteria may help Crohn's disease sufferers. In the meantime, people with Crohn's disease could opt for drinking UHT milk, which has been processed with a technology called UHT (Ultra High Temperature). Its pasteurization temperature is higher than normal and the MAP bacteria have probably been destroyed. And there's always good old soy milk.

If any IBD is suspected, your doctor will send you for either a colonoscopy or a barium X-ray, tests that will give you a good picture of the internal condition of your bowel.

Standard medical treatment for IBD can involve anti-inflammatory drugs like cortisone, as well as antibiotics and even surgery to remove the affected area of the intestine. But more and more sufferers are discovering that diet, exercise, and stress management can minimize or eliminate the need for medication and surgery.

In particular, diet seems to play the most important role in IBD management. Foods to avoid include the usual suspects: sugar and refined carbohydrates, saturated fats, coffee, tea, fried foods, salty foods, alcohol, raw fruit and vegetables, and any foods that you're intolerant to, such as milk or gluten. Things to increase in the diet are fatty acids from fish and oils such as flaxseed, soft fiber (from cooked vegetables or fiber supplements), and probiotics such as acidophilus.

We can safely say that there's a logical pattern emerging: both prevention and treatment of digestive diseases involve smart dietary choices. While this may not seem like rocket science (indeed it appears to be the pretty obvious), it's taken a long time for a lot of people, including many in the medical professions, to embrace this idea of food as therapy.

Appendicitis

At the bottom of the ascending colon, just below the ileocecal valve, is a little worm-like offshoot of the intestine called the appendix. In fact its full name is veriform appendix, the former word meaning worm-like. At one time in human evolution the appendix played a role in digestion, but no more. Instead, it can merely become infected. Doesn't seem right, does it? Oh well.

Appendicitis is, technically, inflammation of the appendix, and when this happens infection follows and the little off-shoot fills with pus. The sufferer will feel pain right around the belly button, which worsens and spreads down the lower right side of the abdomen. An abscess may form in the appendix or it may even burst, spreading the infection through the abdominal cavity and leading to peritonitis. At any point the sufferer may vomit and run a fever.

Treatment for appendicitis is usually surgery to remove the appendix. The condition should be detected and treated early because delayed treatment can lead to life-threatening complications.

Although appendicitis affects around one in every seven people, it is becoming less and less common. In fact, it appears to have been on the decline since the 1930s. The theory is that improved hygiene has changed the profile of our intestinal flora, or bacteria, which is now less prone to infecting the appendix.

Diverticulitis

The colon can develop small protruding pouches that are actually hernias in the muscle wall, called *diverticuli*. They often appear in the descending colon on the left side, which is why they can be associated with pain or tenderness due to inflammation and the presence of a lump or mass on the lower left side of the abdomen. When the pouches become infected it's called *diverticulitis* and can require surgery.

Untreated, diverticuli will become home to unfriendly bacteria that inhibit digestion and eventually lead to toxicity that can affect the immune system. In its most extreme form, diverticulitis can lead to a bowel blockage or even a hole blown through the bowel wall. Ouch. Or the pouches can fill with pus and there might be a high fever with pain that worsens during urination. Any of these situations is obviously a medical emergency and requires treatment in hospital. Diagnosis of diverticulitis is generally made after a barium X-ray or colonoscopy.

In the early stages of the formation of diverticuli there might be no symptoms. Or there might be intermittent pain and even some rectal bleeding. Unquestionably the condition gets worse as we age, and it's estimated that over 60 percent of Americans over 70 have diverticulitis. *Because*—you guessed it—diverticulitis, like so many digestive disorders, is caused by a diet low in fiber and high in refined carbohydrates and saturated fats.

So, prevention involves a high-fiber diet and the reduction of our sugar, carb, and saturated fats consumption to occasional treats. And watch foods that tend to constipate you. As you can imagine, constipation can be a big contributing factor in the formation of diverticuli, so you want to keep things moving at a regular rate.

Gall bladder disease

There are a number of things that can go wrong with the gall bladder, which stores bile and carries waste from the liver. It can become inflamed, swollen, have spasms, scarring, gallstones (which aren't always a problem but certainly *can* be), and it can become backed up if your stomach is producing inadequate stomach acid.

Symptoms of chronic gall bladder problems can include indigestion, burping, bloating, fatigue, headaches, irritability, anxiety, and pale stools. Symptoms of an acute gall bladder attack can include nausea, vomiting, and pain (especially after eating fried or fatty foods), particularly in the upper right of the abdomen, spreading to the shoulder and neck. These symptoms should have you heading straight to the doctor.

Gallstones are hard little chunks that are actually crystallized cholesterol and by-products of red blood cells that build up when the gall bladder fails to empty completely. They can irritate the lining of the gall bladder, especially after you've eaten fatty food, when the gall bladder contracts to deliver bile to the small intestine. This can be painful and should be treated. It's also possible for gallstones to get stuck in the bile duct, potentially leading to jaundice.

The contributors to gall bladder disease include:

- obesity
- high-fat diet
- alcohol abuse
- severe illness
- age (over-forties are at higher risk)
- ethnic and hereditary factors
- diabetes
- cirrhosis of the liver
- inadequate stomach acid.

Many alternative health practitioners also believe that there are more dietary links, such as the over-consumption of refined foods; a low-fiber diet; vitamin and mineral deficiencies; food allergies, intolerance, and sensitivity; rapid weight loss; use of birth control pills and hormone replacement therapy; parasites; lack of exercise, and even skipping breakfast. The huge range of possible causes is one of the reasons you should consult a practitioner if you experience symptoms. You need to have a proper diagnosis to get to the root of the problem.

Gallstones and gall bladder disease can be treated in many ways, from a remedial diet and natural remedies to surgery to have the gall bladder removed. Having the gall bladder removed isn't necessarily as drastic as it sounds, as you can live without one. But if you have gall bladder disease, it's important to learn about all your options so that you can make an educated decision about what sort of treatment will suit you.

It's hard when the so-called experts so often disagree, but that's all the more reason to do your own homework.

Candida

There is probably no more contentious issue relating to digestive disorders than candida. Candida is actually shorthand for a number of terms including *candida albicans, candidiasis* and *candida related complex* (CRC). It might help to start by sorting out what each of them means.

Candida albicans is the scientific term for a common yeast, or single-celled fungus, which is found everywhere on earth and in everyone who lives here. It is a resident in all human intestines and it is one element in healthy bowel ecology. So don't reach for the panic button just because someone says you have "candida."

In contrast, candidiasis is an infection that occurs among people with severely compromised immune systems, such as AIDS and cancer patients. Their normally round yeast cells become elongated and embed themselves in the intestinal wall where they grow wild. Without strong immune systems to act as a barrier, the yeast cells are then absorbed directly into the bloodstream. Candidiasis is diagnosed by a simple blood test or a colonoscopy.

CRC is the condition which—many practitioners claim, but others dispute—occurs when, due to dietary factors, hormonal changes and drug therapy among other things, *candida albicans* grows wild but does not cross into the bloodstream. Instead it supposedly causes inflammation of the bowel lining and produces toxins that can be absorbed back into the bloodstream. The theory is that these toxins can trigger food sensitivities, and combined with the inflammation can cause symptoms of IBS, as well as rectal itching, a white furry tongue, headaches, asthma, chronic fungal infections of the skin and nails, chronic vaginal discharge or vaginitis (thrush), increased pre-menstrual symptoms, depression, and more.

CRC is difficult to diagnose, although some practitioners will do a blood test or check a stool sample. Most doctors believe these tests are meaningless because we all have *candida albicans* in our bodies.

Most conventional medical doctors don't believe that candida overgrowth is a problem in people whose immune systems are reasonably sound. In the opposing corner, many, if not most, naturopaths believe that candida overgrowth is an incredibly common problem that produces a wide range of nasty digestive symptoms. Perhaps the truth lies somewhere in between.

We do know this. Symptoms of so-called CRC can certainly develop after taking antibiotics, and this is because in their zeal to kill off harmful bacteria they kill off *all* bacteria, including healthy intestinal flora like acidophilus and bifidus. Believers in the prevalence of CRC think that a healthy probiotic population keeps the candida population in check. When antibiotics destroy the good flora, there's nothing to stop the candida from growing wild and becoming bad flora. Every woman who has had to use anti-fungal cream or pessaries after coming down with a post-antibiotic case of thrush knows this to be true.

There is also a load of evidence that fungal infections increase just before a woman's period, suggesting that intestinal ecology is affected by reproductive hormones, and there seems to be a causal connection between CRC and birth control pills. Hormone replacement therapy (HRT), steroids, ulcer medication, overindulgence of sweets, alcohol, fruit juice, and refined carbohydrates may also contribute to bowel flora imbalance. There's no question that exposure to radiation and chemotherapy can induce candidiasis. So perhaps less radical drug therapy, such as HRT, steroids etc., really does have an effect, just a less obvious one.

The latest accepted wisdom, even among herbalists and other practitioners of natural therapies, is that CRC has been overdiagnosed in the past. But interestingly, many medical doctors are coming around to the idea that CRC may not be a myth. At least the connection between consuming certain drugs or sweets and the need for a boost in healthy flora is certainly being accepted, whether or not *candida albicans* is involved.

The question remains: what do you do if you suspect you're suffering from CRC?

The first thing you should do is to see a doctor to eliminate more serious problems. Or, you may want to see a herbalist or a naturopath. The important thing is to get some informed guidance about how to treat your symptoms. If CRC is suspected, they'll probably suggest that you go on an "anti-candida diet." This generally involves cutting out sugars, including "natural" sugars like fruits and fruit juices, honey, alcohol, and possibly even milk sugar. The problem is that the idea of cutting out fruit sugars is nonsense, as once in the body they're exactly the same as glucose from starch. In addition to being encouraged to stay away from sugars, you'll be steered clear of foods containing high levels of yeast, such as breads with yeast, mushrooms, cheese, etc., as well as anything containing antibiotics, like many meats.

It's important that you undertake this sort of diet with professional guidance because you'll need to find alternative sources for proteins and calcium if you suddenly cut out all meats and milk. The other thing that will be recommended is that you take high doses of probiotics, and again, you need professional advice about how much and what kinds to take, as they're quite expensive and you don't want it to be a wasted exercise.

It's interesting that so many people do improve if they have symptoms of CRC and go on an anti-candida diet. One study found that people with Crohn's disease improve enormously when they go on an anti-candida diet. But this may not have anything to do with candida itself. Most medical doctors theorize that people's overall health improves simply because replacing sugar, fluffy bread, and alcohol with whole-grain yeast-free bread, more vegetables, and lots of water is better for them, whether or not it affected the population of *candida albicans*. So if you have symptoms, read up on the subject—there are hundreds of books and Web sites devoted to the issue. Listen to the ever-raging debate. And then try what you think makes sense until you find some relief from your symptoms.

Hirschsprung's disease

Hirschsprung's disease (HD) occurs when the last part of the large intestine lacks nerve cells that tell the bowel muscle to push the stool forward. This condition is one that children are born with, so that often infants don't have their first bowel movement when they should. It can be very distressing for both the child and parents.

Sufferers may also vomit bile and have swollen abdomens, as well as intestinal infections. Sometimes symptoms don't appear until later in life, but these sufferers have usually always battled with constipation and possibly anemia.

There are several ways to determine whether someone has HD, including a barium enema and a biopsy, which is the most accurate test. Usually HD is treated with surgery, and recovery will involve changes to the diet, especially a lot of fiber and water.

Colorectal cancer

In 2002, more than 140,000 American were diagnosed with colorectal cancer. Nearly half of them will die from the disease. The tragedy is that many, if not *most* of those cases, could have been prevented, and 95 percent of them would survive if the disease had been caught earlier.

One of the reasons that colorectal cancer doesn't get detected in time is that people are uncomfortable thinking about, talking about, and *doing* anything about their stools. So they fail to go for their yearly (recommended for everyone over age fifty!) fecal occult blood test (FOBT), where the stool is checked for traces of blood. Sometimes people don't even report it to their doctor if they see some blood in their stool. This is how uncomfortable, and capable of denial, some people are when it comes to anything to do with number twos.

Americans are particularly squeamish about looking at their poo. Very few of us do it. There seems to be an archaic and erroneous assumption that people who examine their stools are weird. On the contrary. It's interesting that in many other cultures poo-gazing is not only accepted but also encouraged. Most modern toilets in countries like Japan, Germany, and France have "observation shelves" where the stool falls before being flushed away. Perhaps someday we will be so enlightened.

Another reason for lack of early detection is the fact that in its initial stages, colorectal cancer doesn't produce any symptoms.

Colorectal cancer starts in the cells of the intestinal lining, which reproduce out of control, eventually forming polyps. These polyps, or tumors, are little knobs sticking out from the bowel wall. They are benign at first but if left to thrive they'll become cancerous and eat into the intestinal wall, which is when blood can invade the stool.

There are several factors that contribute to the growth of colorectal cancer. First is simple genetics. If others in your family have had colorectal cancer, you have one chance in eight of getting it too. But by far the main reason that some people get colorectal cancer and others don't appears to be diet. Every study around the world has concluded the same thing: colorectal cancer happens when the diet is low in fiber, high in saturated fats, and high in alcohol consumption. In other words, in "civilized" nations with Western diets. Men get colorectal cancer more often than women, and it's probably because they have diets higher in fat, lower in fiber, and drink more booze. People who get a lot of fiber are protected because fiber feeds the bacteria that produce short-chain fatty acids, which protect the cells that line the bowel. No fiber, no protection. A recent study in Europe showed that a diet based on fruit, vegetables, and whole grains, including oats, almost *halved* the risk of getting colorectal cancer.

There's a higher incidence of colorectal cancer among big meat-eaters, but meat itself may not be the culprit. It's more likely that meat-eaters just don't get enough fruit and veggies that provide antioxidants and fiber for protection. But there's more to the meat connection. It may also be the way meat is cooked that makes it carcinogenic, or cancer-causing. There's evidence to suggest that high temperatures used in barbecuing and frying— enough to blacken the surface of the meat—are culprits. Carcinogenic traces in meat cooked this way are absent in fish, or in meat that is cooked another way. There are also studies that have shown that cooked milk protein contributes to colorectal cancer in animals, so perhaps next time you should think twice about that fifth slice of pizza with all its lovely melted cheese. Especially if this is the third time this week you've had pizza for dinner.

The good news is that there's evidence that fish oils, antioxidant vitamins (D, thiamin, B$_6$, and folic acid) as well as probiotics, especially bifidus, will help protect the intestinal lining against cancerous invasion. And if you get your antioxidants in foods like raw fruits and vegetables, rather than supplements, you'll get more antioxidants directly to the colon.

There's also powerful evidence that regular exercise and maintaining a healthy weight, no matter what your diet, can help lower your colorectal cancer risk. Combined with low-fat, high-fiber foods, you'll be doing everything you can.

So once again, a healthy diet is the key to prevention. But if you're over fifty you should still have an FOBT every year, or a colonoscopy if a member of your family has had colorectal cancer. One in 20 Americans will have the dread disease sometime in their lives. Don't let it be you.

Stomach cancer

Stomach cancer is much less common than colorectal cancer and the dietary link is also less clear. Stomach cancer is much more common in Southeast Asia than in Europe, where the disease is on the decrease, so the typical Western diet doesn't seem to be the culprit. The trigger is uncertain, but there may be environmental factors. The increase may relate to food-borne bacteria in raw, pickled, and smoked foods, which are widely eaten in the region. There is also some indication that a long-term *Helicobacter pylori* infection may be related. Abuse of antacid tablets or liquids might also be a factor in some cases.

Generally the disease develops in the glandular cells of the stomach lining. Untreated, it can spread through the wall of the stomach to the bloodstream and the liver. The symptoms can involve a dull ache and feeling of fullness after even a small amount of food, leading to weight loss. There may also be a burning pain in the upper abdomen.

Stomach cancer usually occurs in people over forty, and can be diagnosed with an endoscopy and sometimes with a barium X-ray. Treatment is effective only if it's caught early, and it may involve removing all or part of the stomach. Afterward the person has to eat very small amounts of food often rather than a few large meals, because the food goes directly from the esophagus to the small intestine. Nutritional supplements are usually needed.

Stomach cancer can also be treated, but not cured, by laser and chemotherapy, which can minimize symptoms and prolong the sufferer's life.

AIDS

Because the immune system is severely suppressed in AIDS sufferers, the digestive system can also be plagued by a variety of ailments. Invading parasites that might not cause a problem in a healthy person can cause massive infection. There can also be chronic diarrhea due to an imbalance of microorganisms as well as other factors, and it's important to work closely with medical practitioners on combination drug and diet therapy. Fiber, probiotics, vitamins, and minerals will also often help to supplement the treatment regime.

Colic

Colic describes any apparent discomfort, usually in infants, caused by spasms somewhere along the digestive tract. Over the centuries, countless home and pharmaceutical remedies have been concocted, many if not most of which don't seem to work. Any parent who has had a baby with colic knows how agonizing it is—for *all* of them. All those tears and whining and apparent pain are terrible to bear, and a cure is so often elusive.

Many associate colic with 666—the "devil's number"—

as it usually occurs from six weeks to six months of age, and is always worse at the "mothering hour" of 6 PM. While this is an amusing coincidence, colic probably has little to do with Satan. Even though it may seem like it at the time.

Colic can be caused by a number of things, all of which appear to result in gas pains. The most obvious short-term trigger is when the baby hasn't been sufficiently "burped" after feeding. It's important to remember that whether they suck from breast or bottle, babies will swallow a fair bit of air when feeding that needs to be released. When you burp the baby, sometimes a bit of milk will come up as well, but this isn't a cause for alarm. If bottle-feeding, make sure the hole in the nipple is big enough, otherwise the baby can be sucking too hard and bring in excessive air. This can also happen when breast-feeding from a mom with retracted nipples. Either way, too much air can get sucked in if the baby simply isn't getting enough food.

If burping the baby doesn't help, there may be another culprit. In breastfed babies it could be something the mom is eating such as broccoli, Brussels sprouts, cabbage, cauliflower, chocolate, cow's milk, onions, or hot and spicy foods. In bottle-fed babies it could be an intolerance to soy milk, cow's milk or additives to the formula. It could also be a vitamin B deficiency, which the doctor can check and then recommend a baby's liquid vitamin B solution to correct.

The problem may also be a structural one. The baby

might have a weak or impaired esophageal valve, possibly due to a hiatus hernia. Or there may be a slight spinal dysfunction brought on by that exciting but cramped trip down the birth canal. If this is the case, gentle craniosacral treatment by a trained osteopath could be the solution.

Hiatus hernia

Hiatus or hiatal hernias are very common and many people have them without suffering any symptoms. A hiatus hernia occurs when the stomach slides too high and presses against other structures, limiting its volume and function. This means that some people get a variety of digestive problems including bad indigestion and reflux.

In some people a hiatus hernia can occur if they're overweight, and losing weight can help. It can also be caused by poor posture, especially a hunched forward pose, and sometimes just correcting the way you sit at your desk can clear things up. Other common sense solutions are: don't drink loads of fluids with meals, don't exercise after you eat, don't overeat, and don't eat right before bed.

Sometimes none of these tricks will work and the best thing to do is visit an osteopath, chiropractor, or remedial massage therapist who will do some soft-tissue manipulation to actually put your stomach back where it's supposed to be. This can bring instant, long-term relief.

Leaky gut syndrome

Leaky gut is a condition associated with other disorders such as celiac disease, and occurs when the intestines become too porous, so that undigested proteins or toxic substances can leak through to the bloodstream and stress the liver and immune system.

Leaky gut can be brought on by parasites, viruses, bacteria, the abuse of NSAIDs, food allergies or intolerance, or even an imbalance between friendly and unfriendly intestinal flora.

If leaky gut is suspected, your doctor can order an intestinal permeability test, which will determine the presence and extent of the condition. Together you'll need to work out the cause of the problem and how to solve it.

Hormonal fluctuations

Because hormonal receptors for estrogen line the intestinal

tract, hormonal swings in women can affect digestion. This is why you can get constipated or sensitive to certain foods just before your period and during pregnancy. The trick here is to anticipate the problem by changing your diet or adding extra water and fiber when you know you'll need them.

Eating disorders

Obviously anorexia and bulimia are incredibly damaging to the whole body, and they have a particularly pernicious effect on the digestive system. If a sufferer is intentionally vomiting food, this means that stomach acid is being repeatedly brought through the mouth, eroding the esophagus, teeth, and gums. The esophageal valve is constantly being challenged to yield the wrong way, which will eventually damage it as well.

Another problem that occurs is that without enough food moving through it to keep its muscles toned, the digestive tract becomes very sluggish, and often bloating and constipation occur. Unfortunately this is the last thing someone with a food disorder wants, and at this point laxatives are frequently resorted to, only making matters worse.

Anyone with an eating disorder needs to get help from both medical and psychiatric practitioners to treat and prevent the many ruinous effects of intentional food deprivation.

Support groups

As with most chronic diseases and conditions, these days there are societies and support groups for sufferers of virtually all digestive problems. From IBS to colon cancer to colic, every disorder has an associated community that helps disseminate information that can help you live with or even overcome the condition. They are usually also on top of the latest breakthroughs and research that can give you hope. Ask your GP for this information or check the Internet. Most groups have their own Web sites, and sometimes it's reassuring just to know that there are others out there in the same boat as you.

Three
Food, Supplements, and Digestion

A couple of thousand years ago when Hippocrates, the father of Western medicine, was practicing, it was widely accepted that food was "functional." In other words, that food could deliver therapeutic benefits. The medicinal properties, particularly of herbs and roots, contributed to an often sophisticated and effective science of health care.

Sadly, in Western societies, this knowledge fell by the wayside with the rise of pharmaceuticals. In the late nineteenth century and most of the twentieth century, doctors and patients overrelied on drugs to cure our ills, including those that affect our digestive systems. Only recently has the notion come back into favor that many diseases can be both treated and prevented by the foods we eat. It's about time.

In the past few decades science has proven that many of our most serious diseases, including colorectal cancer, heart disease, diabetes, and obesity, are caused in part by bad eating habits, or the overconsumption of dysfunctional foods. At the same time they have also discovered that elements in both plant and animal foods can treat and prevent these same diseases. Society once had at least some of this knowledge but forgot it.

Most people are now aware that a diet high in vegetables, fruit, whole grains, and legumes and low in saturated fats and refined carbohydrates is a good diet. But not enough of us are doing enough about it. We know what's right, but we're stuck in the rut of bad eating habits fed by a collaboration between the food and advertising industries that tell us that breakfast cereals full of fats and sugars will turn us into iron men, and fast food is what young, groovy, attractive people gorge on. Well, it's all bullshit.

This isn't a diet book or even a book on general nutrition. There are literally thousands of books on those subjects out there, and it's your job to find the style of diet that works for you, especially in light of whatever personal likes and dislikes, body type, disease, syndrome, allergy, intolerance, or sensitivity you might have. But what this book *will* do is talk specifically about the function of certain foods in terms of your digestive system. This information should be used to complement your overall food plan, and hopefully be of help when your digestive system comes under attack.

Make food welcome

Even if you eat healthy food, it can be hard to digest if you make it unwelcome. If you're rushed or stressed or preoccupied you can ruin even the most wonderful meal because your stomach will be in knots, denied the full attention of your muscles and circulatory system. So try to make the experience of eating a pleasurable and relaxed one, uncompromised by too many distractions. You need to *indulge* in your food.

For meals, create an attractive, comfortable atmosphere. Set the table nicely and take care with the lighting. Put on some good music. Wait to eat when you're hungry—you'll have more digestive juice ready to go to work on incoming food. Eat slowly, chewing thoroughly. Try to avoid drinking icy cold drinks with food, as the cold slows down your digestive system. And don't bolt for the door the second your plate's empty. Sit and let it get happy inside you.

Try to give even your little morning and afternoon snacks a little respect, remembering to de-stress, chew, and relax. A small handful of almonds may sound totally healthy and innocent but if you inhale them, your stomach will make you pay the price for being impatient and lazy with a nice little case of the burps.

Foods that can aid digestion

Many foods can help you maintain a healthy GIT and also treat a mild case of indigestion if it arises. These foods have many wonderful properties that help your body's systems to function well, but detailed below are just those that relate to digestion.

Apples

The old saying "an apple a day keeps the doctor away" has some merit, as this marvelous, inexpensive fruit, available all year round, is high in pectin, a soluble fiber that can help restore healthy levels of friendly bowel microflora.

Aloe vera

A plant whose bitter juice, when heavily diluted, may ease all sorts of symptoms of IBS and other digestive disorders. A powdered form is also available in capsules.

Bananas

Another cheap, easily available fruit that can help soothe gastrointestinal ulcers, especially if the bananas are not overly ripe (bright yellow with brown spots). Also high in fiber.

Cabbage

This vegetable can relieve gas, or in its raw state it can be tossed into the food processor along with a sweet vegetable like carrots for a juice that will soothe an irritated stomach, even one with ulcers.

Celery

In raw or cooked form it's high in fiber and aids digestion.

Essential and nonessential fatty acids

These are omega 3, omega 6, and linoleic acids. Fatty acids are found in foods including fish (especially high levels in ocean fish such as salmon, sardines, and mackerel), leafy green veggies and seaweed, and oils, including safflower, sunflower, evening primrose, flaxseed, hemp, canola, and soy bean. There are tiny amounts in meat and more in game (wild meat). The exciting thing is that fatty acids are great at maintaining the lining of our intestinal tract. Even people who suffer from serious intestinal disorders like Crohn's disease are finding that a diet high in fish (at least four or five servings per week) and vegetables can ease their symptoms enormously. The importance of fish in particular reflects the value of balancing our omega 3 and 6, as most of us have levels that are too high in the latter, while the former can be found in fish.

Figs

Seriously high in fiber. And so delicious!

Garlic

A root that makes the world a better place to live. Not only does it enhance other foods with its flavor—at once devilish and divine—but it has amazing benefits for the digestive system, being antibacterial, antifungal, and anthelmintic (anti-worm!).

Ginger

A root that in raw, dried, or cooked form is great for treating nausea and other digestive upsets, including morning sickness. It's especially palatable in a tea or added to fresh juices. The flavor is hot and zesty, which belies its lovely, soothing effect.

Grapefruit

Like apples, very high in pectin, especially in the white parts that people often don't eat. So eat them.

Licorice tea

Great for treating and preventing mild constipation. And very yummy.

Linseed tea

Using linseed or flaxseeds in a tea is great for healing the bowel or if you suffer from IBS.

Mangoes

Another great high-fiber fruit.

Mint

A plant with several varieties, including spearmint and

peppermint, which can be used in raw or dried form in teas, juices, and sauces. Peppermint in particular is good for nausea, bloating, gas, and IBS. It soothes the belly as it aids digestion.

Miso

Like other cultured foods, it stimulates the growth of friendly intestinal flora. And miso soup is so good for the soul!

Oranges

More high-fiber fruit (and don't avoid the pithy bits where a lot of the good stuff is!).

Pears

Believe it or not, the fruit with the highest level of fiber.

Prunes

These are actually dried plums, and in their whole or juiced form have a profoundly laxative effect. Great for those with constipation.

Pumpkin

Very high in fiber. It's sweet, therefore more kid-friendly than some other high-fiber vegetables, so be sure to include it on family menus.

Seaweed

Ocean vegetables such as agar, nori, and kelp all have important minerals and trace elements that can help maintain digestive function.

Slippery elm

Available in loose powder or capsules, or simply dried for use in teas, the bark of the slippery elm tree is said to soothe irritated GITs and ease symptoms typical of IBS.

Tofu

Another cultured food product that keeps friendly flora thriving.

Yogurt

Milk cultured or fermented with bacteria that can soothe the GIT and balance your intestinal ecology. It's important to check consumer surveys, as there's a huge disparity between brands of yogurt in their varying levels of good bacteria. Some say on the label that they contain live acidophilus and bifidus cultures, but when tested have nearly none. Others are very high, which is what you want. These yogurts can be fine for people with lactose intolerance, as the bacteria actually break down lactose and also produce lactic acid, which alters milk protein, making it less difficult to handle. But only get plain yogurt. The flavored ones contain high levels of sugar, which can reverse the good effects of the microflora. Just add your own fresh fruit, either whole or pureed, and it will be sweet enough.

Food "accessories"

Much has already been said about the damaging effects of diets high in saturated fats, oils, and refined carbohydrates, so there won't be an exploration of how individual foods in those groups can undermine your health. But it may be enlightening to go into more depth about what might be called food "accessories"—things we consume that aren't really food at all in the sense that we don't need or use them to maintain life and growth— and to talk about their effect on your digestive system. We're talking about things like coffee, black tea, artificial sweeteners, and alcohol. For many, it's a case of "can't live with 'em, can't live without 'em." But if you're suffering, you may have to find a way to live without them or at least cut back.

Coffee

Okay, so one or two cups of coffee a day probably aren't going to hurt you. There's even some evidence to suggest that in moderation, coffee (like booze) can actually be *good* for you. Yowza. But if you have a digestive disorder, or you drink it to excess, coffee can be pretty bad news.

A lot of theories and opinions about coffee are controversial and conflicting. Many people have been scared by reports that pesticides used in countries like Colombia where coffee beans are grown is retained and present in the coffee we drink. There is no evidence to support this and it's physically unlikely that pesticides sprayed on the exterior of the plant actually get into the bean. If you're still scared, you can always buy organic coffee.

One of the other suggestions that has coffee drinkers quaking in their boots is that nitrites, a potentially carcinogenic compound, occur naturally in coffee. But nitrite levels in coffee are far lower than those in cured meats like bacon, and vitamins C and E can inhibit the formation of nitrosamines, which is what nitrites become in the body. So if you have a relatively healthy diet you don't have much to worry about.

Coffee does inhibit our uptake of minerals like iron, so it probably shouldn't be consumed with food.

There's conflicting evidence about whether or not coffee stimulates the release of excess digestive juice, and the effects on different people seem to vary. As always, it's important to listen to your own body. If you get an upset stomach after drinking coffee, try going without. Or see if it only happens when you drink it on an empty stomach. Sometimes the solution will be simple.

Generally, in small amounts, coffee is not only not bad for you, there's evidence that it's actually good. Here are some of the nice things about coffee.

- lowers the risk of gallstones and kidney stones
- lowers the risk of colon cancer

- protects against liver disease
- can help asthmatics
- contains antioxidants that help prevent disease
- contrary to common opinion, it doesn't dehydrate.

So don't feel guilty when you order your morning espresso. But if you're drinking three or four or more cups a day, every day, your digestive system among other things (like your sleep patterns) can suffer. By damaging the lining of the intestines, excessive amounts of coffee can prevent nutrients like iron from being absorbed so that vitamin and mineral deficiencies can occur.

And then there are those with certain digestive disorders for whom *no* amount of coffee is a safe thing. If you have gastric ulcers, heartburn, gastritis, colitis, Crohn's disease, stomach or colorectal cancer, or IBS, forget about that cup of joe and open a packet of ginger tea. As hard as it may be to resist, coffee, even decaf, will only make matters worse.

Many coffee drinkers swear by how "regular" coffee makes them, and it certainly contributes to bowel movement. The reason for this is that coffee triggers muscle contraction, but not necessarily in a positive way. The problem is that when the coffee fan stops drinking, that apparently wonderful laxative effect disappears and the bowel has forgotten how to do its job on its own. And the road back can be a very constipated one.

So rely on fiber rather than coffee to keep you regular.

Tea

When we say "tea" we mean the common black tea that most people have along with their newspaper and toast in the morning, not herbal tea. Like coffee, black tea contains caffeine, but we absorb less than we do from coffee because of other buffering chemicals present. The problem with tea in digestive terms is that there's some evidence that it slows down bowel muscle movement, which can lead to constipation. It also may slow down bile production, which makes it harder to digest fats. On the up side, it's rich in antioxidants.

Avoid drinking tea with meals because, like coffee, it inhibits the absorption of minerals such as iron. Again, moderation is the key. A few cups a day, unless you have a digestive disorder, probably won't have any ill effects. But if you're a ten-cups-a-day tea junkie you may be paying a price.

Artificial sweeteners

It doesn't seem fair that when you give up something that's bad for you (excessive sugar) it turns out that its replacement may be even worse! But this is certainly the case with many artificial sweeteners, particularly as they relate to the digestive system.

Artificial sweeteners can be found in sugar-free soft drinks, lollipops, children's medicine, and chewing gum. On the label they're called aspartame, sucralose, mannitol, maltitol, sorbitol, or xylitol. Saccharine was once thought to cause cancer and was banned but became unbanned after these findings were questioned. Once more, the odd dose isn't going to kill you, but repeated exposure can cause stomach and bowel problems including indigestion, bloating, abdominal pain, flatulence, and even diarrhea. Because these additives can't be digested, they travel through the digestive tract to arrive in the bowel where they feed bad bacteria and cause trouble. That's where the bloating and farting come in. Then water floods the bowel and that's when diarrhea strikes.

So if you have any of these symptoms and you're a regular sugarless gum chewer, or "diet" soft drink guzzler, perhaps you should consider a bold move to fresh juices or herbal teas—at least part of the time.

Booze: good news/bad news

Once again, we find that moderation is the magic trick you need to perform to enjoy alcoholic drinks without letting them do you serious damage. Some people find this easier than others, but once you find out *why* moderation is such a good idea maybe it will help you embrace the concept and apply it to your own drinking habits.

The good news is that one or two standard drinks when you finish work and are about to eat can be not only harmless but also good for you. First of all there's the de-stressing factor. A drink can help you unwind incredibly quickly and see the humor instead of the tragedy in the humiliating episode at work that day, or the overdue credit card bill, or your kids' desperate need for the new PlayStation. Stress is one of the biggest contributors to *any* disease but in particular has a lot to answer for when it comes to digestive disorders. If a drink can relax you, that means it relaxes your digestive system. And if your digestive system is relaxed, it's more efficient.

The other thing a drink will do is stimulate your digestive juice, which is why it's a good idea to have a drink before or with a meal. A glass of wine can work the same way as a glass of digestive bitters, but you get the buzz thrown in as well! There is even some evidence that a couple of glasses of wine a day can help prevent an infestation of *Helicobacter pylori*, the bacteria that causes most gastric ulcers. But once more, the effect reverses itself if you exceed the two-drink maximum.

Humans have obviously had alcohol in our diets for a long time, as most of us have specific enzymes for alcohol metabolism. But we can only metabolize so much before the system starts to break down.

As soon as alcohol enters the body it has an effect. First it enters the stomach where about 20 percent of it will be absorbed straight through the stomach wall into the bloodstream. That's why you can feel a drink almost immediately— to a degree alcohol is fat and water soluble and it can penetrate cells easily. And the speed of all this is greater if you have no food in your stomach. If your stomach is empty when you drink, the alcohol will trigger the release of hydrochloric acid. If you drink *a lot* on an empty stomach, the acid can eventually break down the stomach wall's mucous lining. This can lead to gastritis and ulcers, which alcoholics often suffer from.

Once in the bloodstream, alcohol will find its way to the liver, which will attempt to process as much as possible, but at least 5 percent will be carried to the lungs where it will be expelled as you exhale. That's why you can smell alcohol on a drinker's breath, even if they've just had one or two, and that's also how breathalyzers work. They measure the amount of alcohol on your breath and extrapolate how much is in your bloodstream and therefore how much you've actually drunk. Some people (usually ones who've been pulled over for driving in an erratic manner) claim that certain stomach disorders can give false high Breath Alcohol Content (BAC) readings, but there's no real evidence for this.

The alcohol that doesn't get released into the air or absorbed through the stomach wall will continue down through your GIT where it's absorbed in the duodenum. Most of it is metabolized and gives us energy but little in the way of nutrients. Drinking excessively raises the risk of serious digestive diseases, including cancer to the esophagus, stomach, liver, pancreas, and bowel. Everybody seems to know that excessive drinking is bad for the liver, but not as many are aware that it's a big risk factor in colorectal cancer, which is much more common than liver disease.

The other thing that too much booze can do is mess up your movements. And we're not just talking about your breakdancing. After a night of too much imbibing, some people will have diarrhea while others will experience constipation. It can take up to a few days before things are back to normal and you're wondering whether it was worth it.

A word of warning on bubbly. A recent study proved that it's not just your imagination that you get drunk more quickly on champagne, or any sparkling wine. You do. In the study, half the subjects drank still wine and half drank fizzy, with the same alcohol content. Five minutes into the experiment the fizzy drinkers had .54 milligrams of alcohol per milliliter of blood, whereas the still drinkers had .39. The theory is that the bubbles make it easier for the alcohol to permeate the stomach wall, so it gets into the bloodstream faster. This of course explains a lot—like why people get so silly so quickly at weddings and half of them seem to end up falling into the cake on *America's Funniest Home Videos*. Often people put away a half-dozen glasses of the stuff at the reception before the food comes out. Hot tip: eat something before you go to a wedding unless you want to end up a national embarrassment.

Water

There is a lot of confusion about how much water is good for us to drink. Recently the eight glasses (or two liters) per day rule has been challenged, and many of us are wondering what's healthy. It seems that when experts originally came up with the eight glasses formula, they were including the water contained in the foods we eat (especially other beverages, fruit and vegetables), so that we really don't need to drink as much plain water as we thought. On the other hand, different experts still advocate the eight glasses of water *in addition to food* rule.

The fact is that you *can* drink too much water. Excessive amounts of water before, during, and after exercise can cause a severe lack of salt in the blood, leading to illness and even death in rare cases! This condition is actually quite common among inexperienced long-distance and marathon runners. And most of us have heard about cases where excessive fluid intake while taking Ecstasy has led to "internal drowning," causing death. But don't let these facts scare you off water. It remains true that most people could probably benefit from drinking more water than they do, and there are a number of reasons, many pertaining to our digestion.

First of all, we need a healthy water level in the body to produce enough saliva to moisten our food as we chew. Water is a solvent, and it helps nutrients dissolve so that they're easier to break down once they reach the stomach. Once absorbed, water helps blood (which is over 80 percent water) flow against gravity so that nutrients can reach the cells that need them. Water also dilutes and flushes out toxins in the blood. But perhaps the most important benefit in digestive terms is that water softens waste in the bowel so it's easier to move down and out. A lot of people who have suffered chronic constipation find that when they increase their water intake their problem disappears. There's nothing more wonderful than simple solutions.

One of the enduring myths is that coffee and tea will dehydrate you, and you need to counteract the effect by drinking the equivalent amount of water. This is simply not true. You actually retain about *half* their fluid as water, so it's not as dire as you thought. Only a huge amount of caffeine could have a diuretic effect, so load up on the H_2O if you drink buckets of the stuff. Otherwise, relax.

Fiber

There's been a lot of talk about fiber already, and how useful it is in the treatment and prevention of all sorts of digestive disorders, but it really deserves its own section, especially because of recent findings.

According to the latest research, not only does dietary

fiber keep you "regular" and reduce the risk of colorectal cancer, it also seems to lower cholesterol, control blood sugar levels, and may be able to replace some antibiotics! Fiber is truly a wonderful food component.

Water-wise

Drink some water before you exercise

This is important, especially if you break a sweat, to prevent dehydration. Over an extended workout, sip small amounts of water to keep your levels up. And don't forget to rehydrate afterwards as well.

Don't drink too much water

Don't drink more than 16 ounces or excessive amounts of any liquid just before, with, or a while after a meal. You'll be overdiluting your digestive juice, rendering it less effective to break down your food. This can give you a good case of the bloats. On the other hand, you do need some fluid with meals, as it helps food in the stomach become liquid enough to be sent to the small intestine where it can be properly broken down and absorbed. Some health gurus recommend not drinking at all with food, but like so many extreme dietary fads it just doesn't make sense. Water is a solvent and actually helps break down our food.

Have a little lemon or lime in your water

It not only makes it less boring but also aids digestion.

Don't drink ice cold water

Room temperature or even warm water is kinder to your GIT and makes it easier for your gut to do its job.

Beware of sparkling water

Sparkling water can be good for some people and a disaster for others. People with high acid levels seem to react badly to sparkling drinks, as they make enough gas on their own without adding more from the outside. Combining carbonated water with food can create especially unhappy outcomes, unless you like that feeling that you just swallowed a weather balloon. In contrast, others find that sparkling drinks can actually assist digestion and ease bloating as it helps them bring up excess air. Once again, gut reactions are individual, and it's up to you to listen to your body and adjust your habits accordingly.

Drink filtered water

You don't have to go out and spend a fortune and do your back in dragging in expensive imported spring water melted from an iceberg in the Antarctic to get good water. A decent filter will get rid of nasty micro-organisms like giardia and cryptosporidium. It will also filter out chlorine, which can be bad for your healthy intestinal flora because it's antibacterial. It can also deplete the body of vitamins and minerals, and there's evidence to suggest that people who drink a lot of chlorinated water may have a higher risk of bladder and rectal cancer. If you're worried about missing out on fluoride, which most filters get rid of, take fluoride tablets.

Drink enough water to keep your urine pale

One of the simplest ways to figure out whether you're getting enough water is to look at your urine. If it's pale yellow to clear, that's great. It means your body is being hydrated adequately to maintain digestive health and waste disposal. But if your urine is dark yellow to brown, you need to crank up the water intake right away. Dehydration can lead to all sorts of problems, and it's so easy to fix!

The problem is that a lot of people are confused about what kind of fiber is good for them because different types of fiber behave in different ways. Fiber used to be described as either soluble or insoluble, but now they call it dietary or functional. Fiber is basically an indigestible carbohydrate, and the kind you want comes from fruit, vegetables, legumes, beans, and whole grains. It's better to get your fiber from foods than supplements, which can give you just one kind of fiber. Also, fiber that's still part of its source food is actually more effective in doing its job than its isolated counterpart. So it's great if you take psyllium husks to help with your constipation, but don't let that be your only or even your main source of fiber. You should get your fiber from as many different sources as possible.

You should get at least 30 grams of fiber a day. This translates as two pieces of fruit, five servings of vegetables (each serving being half a cup if cooked, one cup if raw) and four servings of bread, cereal, grains, or pasta, all made from whole grains (each serving is the equivalent of two thin slices of bread or a cup of rice.) The average American gets much less fiber than is needed, which is a big reason why the rates of colorectal cancer, diabetes, obesity, and heart disease are so high.

It all makes sense when you understand how fiber works. One of the great things about fiber is that it moves your food more quickly through your GIT when it should, and slows it down when it needs to. For instance, bread made with whole grains will stay in the stomach longer than your average fluffy white bread, which means that nutrients are absorbed more slowly and energy is released to your body gradually rather than in one jolt. This translates as steady rather than surging blood sugar levels and more energy through the day, which also reduces cravings for sugar and carbs with which so many of us fight a losing battle.

Once it gets to the colon, where you don't want what's left to hang around, fiber will give bulk to your waste and stimulate a movement, so it doesn't have time to ferment and create more gas than it needs to. But amazingly, it has the reverse effect on diarrhea. Fiber can actually stop runny stools by soaking up the excess fluid and making the fecal matter swell and slow down long enough for the water to be absorbed across the bowel wall.

Fiber can also absorb excess cholesterol and store it until it's ready to be eliminated with other waste, instead of letting it be reabsorbed into the body. This means that it's good for the cardiovascular and immune systems. It also helps keep women's estrogen levels balanced, so it can help you deal with premenstrual syndrome.

The other spectacular contribution that fiber makes to your digestive and overall health is that it feeds the good bacteria in your lower bowel. The by-products of this union—short-chain fatty acids—are what have antibiotic effects: rather than kill pathogens like gastrointestinal bugs the way that pharmaceutical antibiotics do, they can actually absorb them. At the same time, these by-products also feed the cells that line the bowel wall, guarding against progressive diseases like cancer. And by the way, they minimize antisocial bowel gas. Who would want to live without them?

To put it another way, fiber can help treat and prevent:

- colorectal cancer
- constipation
- diarrhea
- diabetes
- diverticulitis
- gall bladder disease
- gastric ulcers
- heart disease
- hemorrhoids
- inflammatory bowel disease
- intestinal bugs
- irritable bowel syndrome
- obesity
- premenstrual syndrome
- systemic sclerosis
- varicose veins.

So go make yourself a big salad and celebrate a long, healthy life.

To meat or not to meat?

There is a battle constantly being waged between those who believe it is good to eat meat and those who do not. There are many aspects of the issue, including moral and ethical ones that you have to decide for yourself. But how does the question relate to digestion?

When vegetarians argue against the idea of humans eating meat they often cite the fact that we seem to be physically ill-suited to the task. Our teeth are short and relatively flat, like other vegetarian creatures such as horses and cows. Our intestinal tracts are relatively long, once again like our four-legged vegetarian friends who need the length to break down the complex carbohydrates in vegetables, and who will always turn down a cheeseburger in favor of a carrot. Compare these attributes to those of big cats like lions and tigers—avowed meat-only eaters—who have long, sharp teeth for tearing flesh and very short bowels for unloading meat waste quickly, before it has time to ferment and feed unfriendly bacteria. Doesn't sound like us, does it?

While all this may suggest that we are "designed" to be vegetarian, the fact is that we can digest meat, and it's an incredibly good source of protein that we need to live and grow. There is ample evidence from early Homo sapiens that we have been eating meat for at least ten thousand years, and indeed this practice contributed to the growth in our brain size. We probably couldn't have invented game shows without it.

As long as we chew it thoroughly and cook it properly, meat can be nicely broken down by our very powerful stomach acid, pepsin, and pancreatic enzymes, which are well suited to the task. Some might point to the figures regarding colorectal cancer, which suggest that meat eaters are at a higher risk of the disease. While this is true, it's also true that meat eaters often eat fewer vegetables than they should. So the problem may not be too much meat, but too little fiber and antioxidants. Also, our requirements for nutrients such as iron suggest that we need meat. It's very hard to meet these requirements with a vegetarian diet.

The idea of what we're suited or not suited to eat seems to relate more to the region our ancestors came from than to anything else. For example, with many of them being lactose intolerant, Asians and Africans are less suited to consuming cow's milk than Europeans. But it's interesting to note that no race of people, or even individuals, are allergic, intolerant, or even sensitive to meat in the same way. There is no disease like celiac disease (which makes some people unable to digest gluten) that means certain people can't digest meat.

What does seem to be clear is that while we can eat meat, there are better ways to eat and cook it than others. Lean meat is better for us than fatty meat, and charred meat may have carcinogenic properties. Undercooked ground meat can contain E. coli, so burgers should be well done. But more importantly, meat has no fiber or many of the vitamins and minerals that we get from vegetables, fruits, and whole grains, so it should be just a part of our diet, not the mainstay. Alternative sources of protein like fish, nuts, and beans should all be included in a healthy diet. If so, we can enjoy the occasional cheeseburger with a lot less guilt.

Raw food

The latest diet fad is raw food, and its adherents—many of the Hollywood glitterati among them—describe rapturously how eating only uncooked food has changed their lives, making them thinner, more spiritual, more successful celebrities. Restaurants have opened in many major cities that feature only raw food, or food that hasn't been heated above 118°F. The question is: is a raw-food-only diet good for you?

Many in the raw food brigade claim that cooking food kills or neutralizes important nutrients. This is untrue. In the case of vegetables you can overcook them and lose vitamins as well as flavor, but properly cooked vegetables actually allow antioxidants to be better absorbed into the bloodstream. In the case of meat, the cooking process makes the protein easier to digest, and of course, brings out the flavor.

The point is that both cooked and raw foods have special health and digestive benefits. As usual, it's a matter of balance. You don't have to give up cooked food to gain the benefits of eating raw. Juicing a bunch of vegetables and a bit of fruit every day is an incredibly easy and delicious way to get something extra from your food. And it wouldn't hurt to think more about salads as a main course, especially in summer when you don't want to slave over a hot stove anyway. Just remember to include enough protein in the form of beans and nuts to compensate for the lack of a well-done T-bone on your plate.

Supplements

Other books describe the pros and cons of taking vitamin, mineral, and herbal supplements in general health terms, so that's not going to happen here. Except where it relates to the gut. Here are some tips on how supplements interact with your digestive system.

Vitamins and minerals

Amazingly, some people are still unaware that most vitamin and mineral supplements need to be taken with food to be absorbed. Many of us take vitamins first thing in the morning before we've had anything to eat, or maybe just with a cup of coffee or tea. This is a total waste of money. And with what vitamins cost these days, you could be throwing away a down payment on a modest house.

A word about iron. Some people who suffer from bowel disorders have difficulty absorbing iron, so they may need to take iron supplements and/or boost their iron from food sources such as meat and fish. In the short term, some may even need injections. However, iron supplements can cause constipation. And often your stools will become very dark—almost black—from the iron that you're not absorbing.

Don't just start taking iron supplements because you feel a little tired. If you're in doubt, a blood test will tell you whether or not you're short on iron. There may be other causes for your fatigue and you may do more harm than good. Most multivitamins contain several minerals, including iron, that actually compete with each other for uptake by the body, and you may not be absorbing what you need. Also, some people, particularly men, may have too much iron and should avoid supplements altogether. More reasons to get your nutrients from food than food accessories.

Digestive enzymes

At conservative estimates, around 15 percent of us don't produce enough digestive enzymes on our own to digest our food properly. This might be caused by aging, stress, poor diet, suppressed immune system, zinc deficiency, or exposure to dietary and environmental toxins. Symptoms may include burping, bloating, indigestion, nausea, whitish coated tongue, muscle cramps, loose stools, weak nails, anemia, skin problems, and possibly asthma, although these can also be caused by other things and some of these connections are disputed.

Because of the many variables that may be involved, it's important not to self-diagnose inadequate digestive enzymes. With the help of your healthcare practitioner, you need to get to the root of the problem and stop it at its source if you can. To relieve your symptoms in the short term, your practitioner may recommend that you take digestive enzyme supplements that are combined with minerals and herbs in tablet form. But don't take them indefinitely or if they trigger a burning sensation.

Calcium

It's not just for strong bones. Recent research has found that calcium plays a significant role in preventing some bacterial infections of the GIT, including salmonella and E. coli, and it may even help to prevent colorectal cancer. The way calcium does this is by feeding friendly intestinal flora like acidophilus (which fights the infection), and also by making waste products in the colon more soluble and easier to eliminate. The best way to get your calcium is from food sources like milk and yogurt, but you can also take supplements. The recommended daily level is about 800 milligrams per day, up to 1200 milligrams where there is a risk of osteoporosis. Recent studies have shown that up to 2500 milligrams a day may give even more protection and still be safe, although it could interfere with the absorption of other minerals. As with any supplement, talk to your practitioner about dosages and how calcium may interact with other drugs or supplements you're taking.

Herbs

For thousands of years societies all over the world have successfully treated digestive disorders with herbs. Often this therapeutic skill was in the hands of a shaman or medicine man or woman who was the most revered member of the community. A lot of societies lost these skills when they became "civilized," and women who knew their fenugreek from their fennel were often burned at the stake as witches. Well, thank goodness that phase of religious enlightenment is over and herbs have come back into fashion as important therapeutic tools.

If you have a digestive disorder and you're interested in treating it with herbs, you should see a trained herbalist. Often this person will also be a naturopath, an acupuncturist, a nutritionist, a homeopath, a practitioner of Traditional Chinese Medicine (TCM), or even a medical doctor. Herbs have amazing properties relevant for digestive disorders and can be antispasmodic, anti-inflammatory, laxative, muscle relaxing, emotionally relaxing, and stimulating to the digestive and circulatory systems. Often herbs can replace a pharmaceutical medication like NSAIDs that can be contributing to your digestive problem.

You might need to take certain herbs as a tea or in a tonic, or as a dry powder mixed in water. If you go this route, stick with the recommended remedy long enough to let it work. Generally, herbal remedies have a cumulative effect and take longer to work than pharmacy products. Sometimes they may take weeks, or even months. And don't back off just because the herbs taste foul. Since when was medicine supposed to taste good?

You can also get various herbal tonics and tablets at your local health food store that can treat a variety of digestive symptoms. Some of the herbs often included in these treatments are: ginger, golden seal, capsicum, fennel, fenugreek, licorice, peppermint, raspberry, slippery elm, and wild yam. But don't mess around with herbal treatments without guidance. They have very powerful properties that may negatively interact with other medications such as anticancer or antipsychotic drugs, and they may affect other conditions you have, including pregnancy, allergies, epilepsy, schizophrenia, or if you've had an organ transplant. Always talk to an expert first.

Probiotics and prebiotics

These have been mentioned in passing, but definitely deserve to be expanded on. The word "probiotic" is derived from Greek, meaning "for life." Probiotics are beneficial bacteria that can be consumed with food, like yogurt, or taken as a supplement in either powdered or encapsulated form. The use of probiotics is nothing new. People along the eastern Mediterranean and parts of Asia have used fermented dairy products like yogurt for centuries, knowing them to be good for overall health.

What probiotics do is repopulate the gut, which needs friendly flora in high numbers to maintain digestive health. Almost all intestinal bacteria live in the colon where they can have a mass approaching two pounds, so they collectively almost operate as an organ! There are many types of probiotic bacteria, but you've probably heard of lactobacillus acidophilus and bifidobacteria—in shorthand often referred to as lactobacillus or acidophilus, and bifidus.

Prebiotics are nondigestible food ingredients that stimulate the growth and function of friendly flora. Perhaps the most exciting prebiotics—oligosaccharides—are found in foods such as asparagus, bananas, beans, milk, wheat, and yogurt. Prebiotics have antibacterial properties, and they feed and maintain our beneficial bacteria population. Many probiotic powders and capsules are now being packaged together with prebiotics. This enticing cocktail is called symbiotics and can help to keep your gut working like a well-oiled machine.

But what exactly do they do?

Your many varieties of friendly flora perform an impressive array of digestive tasks. They break down carbohydrates in the bowel into short-chain fatty acids that supply energy. They help to stimulate the production of digestive enzymes, minimizing gas and bloating. They prevent constipation. They appear to improve the absorption of minerals. They block the production of nitrosamines, those nasty carcinogenic byproducts of processed meats like bacon and hot dogs. They help digest fats and lower cholesterol, therefore reducing the risk of heart disease. They inhibit the overgrowth of yeasts like candida albicans. They can even work like natural antibiotics, enhancing our immune systems. They actually produce some B vitamins and vitamin K, as well as lactase, the enzyme that helps digest milk sugar. You definitely want to keep your friendly intestinal flora happy and flourishing.

The problem is that there are a lot of things that can kill off our good flora. The ecology of our GIT is very sensitive to change, and often the bad bacteria or flora can get the upper hand on the good flora. This is called dysbiosis, and it can be caused by taking drugs such as antibiotics and steroids. It can also be triggered by intestinal infections, hormone swings, stress, too much sugar and other dietary imbalances, drinking a lot of tap water high in chlorine, X-rays, radiotherapy, constipation, diarrhea, eating food treated with pesticides, herbicides, fungicides, and eating meats containing antibiotics. And then there's aging. The older we get the more our friendly flora decrease in numbers and potentially harmful bacteria increase. This, along with the need for reading glasses, is another of the many charming aspects of growing old.

Dysbiosis can lead to mild symptoms like bloating, or serious symptoms like inadequate nutrient absorption, and contributes to all the other diseases like colorectal cancer that healthy flora help to prevent.

So, when dysbiosis occurs you need to replace the lost

friendly flora, and just eating yogurt that contains acidophilus every morning isn't going to do it. You will need to
take probiotic supplements available at health food stores.
They need to be refrigerated or the bacteria will become
inert. You can take them either in powdered form, mixed with
water, or in capsules. There are conflicting theories as to
when is the best time to take them. Many doctors and indeed
the manufacturers of probiotics suggest that the powdered
form should be taken in a glass of water at least half an hour
before breakfast as they work best on a GIT as empty as possible. Other practitioners believe that they should be taken
with food, which can buffer the friendly flora from the
effects of stomach acid. This is why it's perhaps best to use
the encapsulated form, as the capsule will protect what's
inside and you can take it any time.

The amounts and varieties you take depend on your particular problem, which is why you should consult a practitioner before forking over your hard-earned dollars. Probiotic
and prebiotic supplements are expensive, and like any therapeutic supplement they shouldn't be taken casually or care-
lessly. To get a reading of the levels of friendly and unfriendly
bacteria your stools can be tested, although this won't tell you
which bacteria are present in the ascending colon.

More and more studies confirm that probiotics, prebiotics, and symbiotic supplements can help treat a huge variety
of digestive diseases. No matter what your disorder, if it has

anything to do with the gut you should talk to your doctor about probiotic therapy.

Benefits of probiotics and prebiotics

- anti-tumor properties
- cholesterol lowering
- improved overall digestion
- relief from constipation
- treatment of traveler's diarrhea
- stimulation of the immune system
- improved resistance to gut infections such as food poisoning
- vitamin production
- relief from symptoms of IBS
- possible alleviation of symptoms of chronic fatigue syndrome

Four
Drugs and Digestion

*E*verything we ingest we have to digest, and that includes drugs. Many of us think of drugs—both medicinal and recreational—as something we take and they go straight into the bloodstream and get to work, unlike food. But it's not as simple as that. Depending on the drug, it can interact with your digestive system in many ways. An awareness of these could be important.

There are many different kinds of drugs on the market designed to treat digestive disorders, and most of them do what they say they do. Some of them don't. Some of them have side effects that can actually make matters worse, and some don't. Some are safe to take for a short period but not for long. The important thing to remember when taking any kind of drug, whether it's a seemingly innocent over-the-counter medication or a prescription drug, is that you should ask your doctor or pharmacist about side effects and possible problems or complications arising from interaction with other drugs or supplements you're taking. Practitioners don't always think to ask you about those things, and it's not their job anyway. These vital pieces of information are up to you to put together.

And read the label. It might seem boring but it could tell you something you need to know. And don't freak out at all the things they say could happen: Negative side effects are a bit like terrorism—you need to be alert, not alarmed.

Antibiotics

Antibiotics are truly wonder drugs, and we should all be happy we are living in a time and a place where we have access to medications that can kill infections that used to kill people, and still do in many countries. In the case of digestive disorders, antibiotics are used for a variety of complaints, including ulcers and intestinal parasites. If you're prescribed antibiotics, make sure you take the whole course. In some cases where your infection is persistent (very common when bacteria invade the GIT) you'll need to take a second course.

Whether you take antibiotics for an intestinal problem or for anything else, you need to repopulate your intestinal tract with friendly flora after the course is finished. This was mentioned in the section on probiotics, but it's so important that it's worth nagging you about. Antibiotics taken to wipe out bad bacteria will also wipe out good bacteria. This applies whether the antibiotics you take are for pneumonia or for *Helicobacter pylori*. To restore ecological balance to your belly and ensure a digestive system in good working order for the future, take probiotics in either powder or capsule form and ask the supplier or your practitioner about dosages. You'll want to take more than the recommended minimum on the label, which usually refers merely to a maintenance dose.

Some antibiotics can also destroy digestive enzymes in the small intestine, therefore making it hard to absorb nutrients. Discuss with your doctor ways of counteracting this effect if your prescription may cause this problem.

Acid suppressants and antacids

If your stomach is producing too much acid, or you need to limit the amount of gastric juice you make while you're recovering from such disorders as ulcers, you may need to take something to suppress the acid. Some acid suppressants are available over the counter, and others are prescription only. Most of these have no side effects, but some can cause drowsiness, headaches, or a rash. You need to talk to your doctor or pharmacist about these drugs, because they can also affect the way other common prescription medications are processed by the liver. As usual, the message is "buyer beware."

Over-the-counter antacids (in tablet or liquid form) work by chemically neutralizing your gastric juice. Be careful because the ones with aluminum can make you constipated, and the ones with magnesium can give you diarrhea. Also, a lot of antacids contain salt, which can be bad for people with heart or kidney disease or high blood pressure. In any case, don't take them for long periods. There is some evidence that aluminum can be absorbed into the bones and the brain, contributing to osteoporosis and possibly Alzheimer's disease. Once more, the idea is that drugs like this can only treat symptoms, so ultimately you need to solve the problem that leads to the symptoms. Just treating symptoms can be dangerous.

Antispasmodics and muscle relaxers

Often recommended for treatment of diarrhea associated with IBS, antispasmodics can also help to release trapped wind and the pain that can come with it. But because they reduce fluid secretions, they can also cause dry, itchy skin and even a dry cough as well as other possible side effects.

Your doctor may prescribe muscle relaxers, which will let the bowel muscle let go of the spasm that's causing the constant flow of water and waste. The only problem here (aside from your not being able to operate heavy machinery . . . like a hair dryer) is that the muscles become so relaxed that they forget all about peristalsis and you might become constipated.

Opioid analgesics

Another way to get the bowel muscles to stop contracting and causing diarrhea is through opioid analgesics. These include codeine and morphine, and are strictly for short-term use. Long-term use will lead to addiction and a ruined liver, bad breath, no friends, and so on. Well, that may be an exaggeration, but you get the idea. They're generally only prescribed when your diarrhea is caused by a bacterial infection, rather than IBS. And they can actually make muscle tension worse if caused by anxiety.

The way opioid analgesics work is that they tell the brain to tell the muscles to stop moving. The potential problem, once again, is constipation. Even small amounts of codeine available in painkillers without a prescription (usually mixed with paracetamol) can cause constipation, so if you need to take even a couple of codeine and tend toward constipation, bulk up on your water and fiber for the duration.

Alginate

Alginate can be a good treatment for reflux, as it floats on top of whatever is in your stomach, so that if you bring some back up it will soothe the lining of the esophagus and protect against your stomach acid. Usually drugs with alginate (derived from seaweed) also contain an antacid.

Laxatives

There are several different kinds of laxatives and none should be used regularly because, as we talked about earlier, it's easy to become dependent and your bowel will forget how to do its job without them. Some laxatives, like those made with senna, work by irritating the lining of the bowel to trigger a movement. Not only is dependency a problem with these, but permanent damage to the bowel wall can occur if this type of irritation becomes a regular thing.

Other laxatives, like epsom salts, draw water into the bowel, and others are fecal softeners, which can be taken orally or as suppositories. Once more, none of these solutions is preferable to regularity induced by a high-fiber diet and regular exercise.

If you have been taking laxatives for a long time, stop and change your diet but also take a long course of probiotics, as the friendly flora will have been stripped from your intestines. Probiotics will also help to keep you regular.

Anti-inflammatories

Steroidal anti-inflammatories may be prescribed for inflammation due to ulcers caused by colitis and Crohn's disease and can reduce pain, swelling, and even leakage. However, steroids shouldn't be taken indefinitely and can lead to all the terrible side effects you've probably heard about associated with the drugs, including easy bruising, capillary breakdown, muscle wasting, protein deficiency, diabetes, and more.

Aminosalicylates also have anti-inflammatory properties by inhibiting bacterial growth and enzyme activity that cause ulcers. But once again, these are only for short-term use.

Antidepressants and tranquillizers

If your digestive problems like IBS are primarily caused by anxiety, your doctor may recommend antidepressants or tranquillizers. These days, antidepressants are prescribed much more often than tranquillizers and are intended for long-term use. The widespread popularity among doctors and patients of drugs like Prozac certainly attests to the fact that for a lot of people they work. But they can have side effects such as negative food interactions, eating disorders, headaches, insomnia, and nausea. This is still an area awash in controversy, but there is some evidence that antidepressants can also lead to uncharacteristic and even psychotic behavior. Obviously at the first sign of anything like this you should stop taking the drug, see your doctor, and consider enrolling in a meditation class or pursuing any number of ways to reduce and control stress.

Having more of a sedative effect than antidepressants, tranquillizers like Valium are intended only for short-term or intermittent use and are addictive. They can also cause constipation, clumsiness, fuzziness, short-term memory loss, and hangovers. Go there with extreme caution.

Nonsteroidal anti-inflammatory drugs (NSAIDs)

The most common and popular NSAID is aspirin, a mild painkiller that may do serious harm to your stomach if taken for long periods. NSAIDs reduce inflammation by lowering your production of chemicals called prostaglandins. The problem is that while prostaglandins can cause inflammation in the joints, they also protect the stomach against its own acid. So with less prostaglandin, gastric juice can eat away at the stomach lining causing indigestion and eventually even ulcers.

Ibuprofen, another NSAID available over the counter, is a little gentler on the stomach, but it's still a smart idea to take it with food to minimize the potential damage.

If you need to take anti-inflammatories for a long time you may also want to take another drug to protect your tummy, but first consult your doctor, as the more drugs you take the more chances there are for negative interactions and side effects.

Stronger anti-inflammatories available by prescription can also hurt your digestive system, so if you have to take them for a while, it might be worth taking them as suppositories. Not the ideal alternative, but better than a bleeding ulcer.

Lipase inhibitors

In light of our current pandemic of obesity, drugs that control fat uptake are bound to be popular. Note that we say "uptake," not "intake." Your doctor can prescribe a drug called a lipase inhibitor that actually reduces the amount of fat that you absorb from your food. The way it works is that it prevents some fat from crossing the intestinal wall into the bloodstream.

But there are a few problems with this arrangement. First, it would obviously be better to take in less fat in the first place. For your overall health, food volume should be comprised of fruits, vegetables, lean protein, and fiber more than with fats. Also, lipase inhibitors can only reduce fat uptake by one-third. And the fat that isn't absorbed passes through to the colon undigested. If too much fat is eaten the colon can't cope, and anal leakage or diarrhea can occur. This is a very high price to pay. Lipase inhibitors should be used only as a last resort, and only while other weight loss measures are being taken at the same time.

Marijuana

It's a well-documented fact that marijuana is an effective treatment for nausea associated with chemotherapy. For this purpose there are also synthetic equivalents of its active ingredient, tetrahydrocannabinol (THC), that don't make you stoned. Marijuana is also effective for HIV/AIDS sufferers who are experiencing a loss of appetite. If you fall into any of these categories, talk to your doctor about whether marijuana would be a good solution for you.

Smoking

As if the prospect of lung cancer, heart disease, blindness (from macular degeneration), and wrinkles weren't enough to put you off cigarettes, there are also serious digestive complications that can be caused by smoking.

The impact of smoking on your GIT is insidious and works in two ways. First, it stimulates the release of digestive acid in the stomach, and since you're not eating this just means all that acid is churning around with nothing to do but work away on the stomach wall. This is how smoking can contribute to the emergence of gastric ulcers, and can make already existing ulcers a lot worse. Short of causing ulcers, this effect can give you heartburn (reflux).

The second thing smoking does is make small blood vessels constrict, shutting off the blood supply to the stomach. The worst thing you can do is light up right after a meal—

often when you really crave a smoke—because you need a free-flowing blood supply to help feed the stomach muscles and absorb nutrients. What can happen is reduced absorption of things like vitamins and minerals. Ultimately this restriction of the blood supply to the digestive system can be a factor in conditions including ulcers, colitis, IBS, and stomach and colorectal cancer. So if you haven't gotten the message yet, perhaps the idea of having to use a colostomy bag for the rest of your life will help you kick the habit.

Many smokers have noticed that even a puff or two on a cigarette can stimulate a bowel movement. This is because the nicotine triggers a contraction in the colon, and while the immediate outcome may be satisfying, the long-term effects are not.

Five
Stress and Digestion

S tress isn't the problem. The problem is the way we react to it. And the way most people react to it can lead to all sorts of diseases, especially those that affect your digestive system. The thing is that stress isn't going to go away. There will always be dickheads, situations at work, traffic jams, and bad pop songs in your life that have the potential to drive you crazy and make you anxious. This is why you have to take responsibility for your stress management. You can't always control the things that stress you, but you can control how you handle them.

The reason that stress is so hard on our digestive systems is chemical. When we experience fear or anger, the hormones adrenaline and noradrenaline are released as part of our ancient fight-or-flight game plan. What they do is first stimulate the digestive muscles to dump their contents before shutting them down. This is why someone can literally be "scared shitless." And why you might feel the urgent need to visit the toilet just before you have to deliver a speech to a live audience. Anyway, after the signal to evacuate (your bowels as well as the room) come more signals. In response to these signals, your blood vessels are constricted, secretion of fluid is stopped (that's what gives you dry mouth when you're nervous or afraid) and movement in the intestinal tract is stopped. Effectively, digestive activity shuts down. Even the ability to empty the bladder is inhibited.

So if you have food being broken down when you're under stress, you'll absorb less of the nutrients and everything will come to a standstill. It's easy to see how experiencing stress can contribute to all sorts of digestive trouble, from mild indigestion to IBS to constipation to cancer. Now that you know all this, the trick is to stop your body from getting tied up in knots every time the light turns red.

The good news is that you have a magnificent range of choices when it comes to stress management techniques. And most of them won't cost you a cent. All they'll cost you is a little bit of time in exchange for general good health and perhaps even the alleviation of symptoms that have been bothering you for years!

Visualization

To visualize simply means to imagine that you're seeing something. The amazing thing is that 65 percent of the area of your brain that's used to actually see is also used to visualize. What this means is that when you imagine you're seeing something, your brain acts as if you really are, and will send out signals to the rest of the body accordingly. For example, it's been demonstrated that if someone merely imagines that she's lifting heavy weights, there is significant muscle activity in the arms, shoulders, and abdominals.

There are many scientific studies that support the claim that mental visualization can help in the treatment of and recovery from all kinds of physical diseases. This is particularly true with digestive disorders, which are so deeply affected by stress and emotions.

So, if you have a particular digestive problem, try picturing it in your mind and watch it heal. For example, if you're constipated, imagine the muscles of the wall of the colon and picture them having those healthy wave-like motions. If you focus on your GIT this way, you can help it work and heal.

Or, you may not want to focus directly on your problem, but address the stress associated with it. In this case, you merely need to lie or sit in a comfortable position, close your eyes, and imagine yourself in a safe, peaceful, beautiful place. For you, it might be in a deep bath in a luxurious bathroom.

Or having a massage. Or lying in a hammock on a beach while being fanned by Viggo Mortensen. Whatever the image is, it will stimulate subtle muscular movements that will gradually relax your body and your mind. This is a pleasant, easy way to keep stress from eating you alive.

Meditation

More and more, the medical and scientific establishment is recognizing the therapeutic benefits of something that for many people used to be associated only with exotic religions. GPs now often refer patients to meditation courses, and oncologists regularly recommend meditation as part of cancer patients' treatment and recovery program. All this because studies have found that meditation can alleviate symptoms of IBS, ulcers, and even cancer, and it certainly helps in pain management, including pain from intestinal diseases and surgery.

The following experiment was performed at an American university to illustrate the effectiveness of meditation as a stress management tool. While a Buddhist monk was meditating, researchers set off an explosive sound equivalent to a gunshot right next to the monk's ear, and his heart rate and blood pressure actually decreased. And he didn't even flinch.

Well, you don't have to be a Buddhist monk to get health benefits out of regular meditation, but it helps if you know what you're doing. This is why it's good to learn basic techniques from someone with the proper training. You don't have to go to classes every week. But in the early stages it's good to get sufficient guidance so you know what you're doing and you don't waste time.

Basically, meditation is a state of extreme relaxation achieved through rhythmic breathing and the clearing of the mind, often with the aid of visualization and a mantra, or a repeated word or phrase. Once you get the hang of it, you can meditate even for a few minutes at a time and get some benefit, especially if you need some quick stress relief. For example, some deep breathing and mental clarity on your way to the podium to deliver that big speech or in the elevator on your way to a job interview can help keep your stomach and bowel from tightening into a knot it won't want to get out of. The point is that meditation is an incredibly handy tool to help us survive with our health intact in the modern world.

There are many ways of meditating and you need to find the style that suits you. Delve into the hundreds of Web sites, books, audiotapes, or classes devoted to the subject and you'll get an idea of what's on offer. Ultimately, like everything else, the technique you choose needs to be right for you.

Aromatherapy

The soothing, healing properties of plant extracts have been known since the ancient Egyptians used them, but they've come back in a big way in the last couple of decades. Aromatherapy involves the use of different essential oils that are derived at the plants' maturity for greatest potency. The oils can be used in different ways—burned, in the bath, inhaled in a steam, or massaged into the skin. Especially as a way to manage stress, aromatherapy is simple, inexpensive, and pleasurable.

Some of the essential oils that are said to be particularly good for relaxation are:

- bergamot
- chamomile
- clary sage
- frankincense
- jasmine
- lavender
- marjoram
- neroli
- peppermint
- rose
- sandalwood
- ylang ylang.

There are a lot more essential oils that you can learn about through books or from your local health food store. But be aware that you shouldn't use them during pregnancy without the advice of a professional, as there are a few that can cause miscarriage. (At least that shows how much of an effect they can have!) As with everything else, which oils are best for you depends on personal taste. So experiment, relax, and enjoy.

Medication

Antidepressants have already been talked about, but in the discussion of stress management it's important to differentiate between stress and depression. Drugs such as Prozac are for people with clinical depression and those who suffer from anxiety, posttraumatic stress disorder, and other similar conditions, not for people who are experiencing the inevitable and universal effects of everyday stress. All drugs have side effects, and it's always better to find natural solutions, especially in the long term. So don't insist that your GP write you a prescription for antidepressants just because stress sometimes gets to you. Talk to him or her about your other options, and explore them intelligently. Quick fixes almost always have unwanted repercussions, and often what appears to be a quick fix at first turns out to be merely an illusion.

Tranquilizers actually make more sense for the short-term treatment of unmanageable stress, but you need to resist the temptation to take them like vitamins, along with your yogurt and coffee at breakfast.

Easy ways to stress less

Work to live, don't live to work

Don't imagine that your job is the most important thing in your life. If it is, the pressures of work might really be getting to you, and if they are, you're losing. So get a life. Spend time with your family, friends, do some volunteer work, get a hobby, read books, take up the tango, but whatever you do, remember that what we do for a pay-check does not constitute the meaning of life.

Talk to your friends

This simple act is one that we sometimes neglect when getting on with our busy lives. But we shouldn't forget that keeping our problems bottled up inside can literally turn them against our own digestive system. So always make time to hang out with friends over a cup of tea or a pint of beer. Even if you don't get any useful advice— or even talk directly about what's bugging you—the social interaction is sometimes enough to bring you back from the brink of stress burnout.

Exercise

Any form of physical exercise that you can do safely will help you deal with stress. You'll feel better, breathe easier, and be a calmer person if you get some exercise at least three or four times a week.

Sleep

Many, if not most of us, are sleep deprived. This will have consequences on both physical and mental health. If you have to get up early, make sure you're in bed early. If you feel the urge and you can possibly get away with them, take naps. The siesta is arguably the most civilized thing southern Europe has to offer, but unfortunately this wonderful custom didn't really make the trip to America with many of its immigrants. But there are many of us secret nappers out there. So join the club and give your body the time to rest and heal so that stress doesn't kill you.

Practitioners, Tests, and Digestive Disorders

Six

F or many people with digestive disorders, the first practitioner they visit will be their general practitioner, or general medical doctor (GP). To maximize your chances of being cured, it's important to have the right attitude when making this visit. You need to realize that your doctor needs your help if he or she is to figure out what's wrong with you and how to fix it. Ultimately, all relationships with practitioners should be collaborative. Unless you're willing to put in as much effort as they are you might as well not bother.

To make this collaboration as successful as possible, make sure you're prepared. Before your visit:

- Gather any medical records that might be relevant, including X-rays, blood test results, etc.
- Write a list of your symptoms as well as the approximate dates they appeared.
- Write a list of any medicines, vitamins, minerals, and herbs you're taking.
- Write down all your questions.

During your visit:

- Refer to your lists and be completely honest. The color of your poo and the frequency of your motions may not seem like polite conversation, but these things may be exactly what your doctor needs to hear about to make a proper diagnosis. What may be strange and embarrassing to you, your doctor has heard a hundred times before. So chill out.
- Write down your doctor's advice so you don't forget something important later, like the fact that you need to stop drinking fourteen cups of coffee a day.
- Ask questions. There's no such thing as a stupid question, only stupid answers. So ask away—your practitioner is trained to deliver smart answers.

Following these handy hints will help you get the most out of your visit to the doctor. And they'll empower you to help heal yourself once the visit is over.

All GPs have slightly different styles, but they'll all start by asking for a medical history, if they don't already have one for you. After you discuss your current symptoms—and get through your lists—the doctor will do a physical examination.

Afterward you'll be advised on a course of action. This may involve immediate treatment of your symptoms with drug therapy and/or nutritional advice, or you may be referred for tests. The doctor may take some blood for testing as well. *Or*, you may be referred to a specialist doctor or a complementary therapist as described later.

It may be useful to know that GPs are required to do only a minimal course in nutrition while at medical school. But some GPs have taken it on themselves to further study the science of nutrition and dietetics and incorporate more food-based treatments to help their patients deal with digestive disorders. Others have not. It's up to you to discover what degree of nutritional training your GP has and what his or her philosophy is about food as therapy. Ultimately you want a GP who you can work with and who will help you heal yourself.

Diagnostic tests

When you visit your GP with a digestive complaint that's been bothering you for a while it's likely that he or she will order some kind of test or tests to determine the cause of your symptoms. Sometimes this is mostly precautionary, and the tests are just needed to eliminate more serious ailments than the GP really suspects. But it's always better to be safe than sorry, so it's important to comply with their recommendations.

Blood test

The blood reveals a huge amount of information about the inner workings of the body, in particular about the digestive system. If your doctor suspects you may have an ulcer or the presence of *Helicobacter pylori*, a blood test can show whether or not you have the antibodies that your body would have produced to fight the bacteria. Your GP may take the blood or you may need to go to a pathology lab. In either case, you will have results back in a few days. Although not 100 percent accurate, a blood test in most cases can also reveal whether a patient has celiac disease. This test will be relied on when more invasive tests are decided against.

A blood test can accurately show levels of some but not all vitamins and minerals, therefore whether a digestive disorder has led to a nutritional deficiency.

Your blood will also reveal different aspects of your liver and pancreatic function, which are such essential parts of the digestive process. If there is a breakdown in any of these systems your blood will tell all.

Ultrasound

Ultrasound is a scanning technique that can generate images that distinguish between different tissues inside the body. It's a simple, totally painless procedure, whereby the patient lies on a bed while a radiographer or radiologist puts a lubricating gel on the skin. Then he or she holds a horizontal bar that emits inaudible sound waves onto the area to be investigated and drags it gently across the skin. The internal image will appear simultaneously on a monitor (like a TV screen). The image on the screen is actually the shape of the sound waves bouncing off your internal organs. You need to fast from both food and fluids before an ultrasound so that your organs are empty and therefore more defined.

An ultrasound scan can reveal the size and shape of your stomach, liver, gall bladder, pancreas, and spleen, all of which contribute to the overall picture of your digestive health. In particular, ultrasounds are the best test for gall bladder disease, as any gallstones present will show up clearly, as will as any thickening of the gall bladder wall or blockage of the bile ducts.

Endoscopy

A wonderful high-tech test, the endoscopy is administered by a gastroenterologist to diagnose a variety of digestive diseases.

Performed in a hospital or speciality clinic, an endoscopy involves the use of a thin, flexible tube containing a fiberoptic video camera to examine your gastrointestinal tract. When used to examine the upper GIT, including the esophagus, stomach, duodenum, and the upper section of the small bowel, an endoscopy can also be called a gastroscopy.

After the patient has been sedated, the endoscope is inserted via the mouth and feeds the images directly to a video screen, which the doctor observes to monitor the search. Ulcers or gastritis associated with *Helicobacter pylori* will be visible. At this point a biopsy can also be taken to determine the presence of *Helicobacter pylori*, as well as celiac disease and other problems related to poor absorption of nutrients. The endoscope can also suck up a sample of stomach juice for analysis. The possibility of stomach or esophageal cancer, or other conditions of the esophagus, can also be eliminated with this test.

Colonoscopy, enteroscopy, sigmoidoscopy, and proctoscopy are the tests where an endoscope or an enteroscope is used to examine the lower gastrointestinal tract to varying depths depending on the patient's condition, and is inserted through the anus. Similar to an endoscopy, these also involve the taking of tissue samples. These tests can detect a host of lower GIT disorders including celiac disease, ulcerative colitis, Crohn's disease, colorectal cancer, precancerous polyps, nutrient malabsorption, and other conditions. Before any of these tests are done you'll need to clear your colon of any waste material, and your doctor will advise you on how to take strong laxative solutions for this purpose.

Once again, during these procedures the patient doesn't feel a thing as he or she is completely sedated, and there is no postprocedural discomfort. With an endoscopy there may be some soreness in the throat and, as with all invasive procedures, there are some risks of tearing or reaction to the anesthetic, but they are *very* small.

To diagnose problems in the liver, gall bladder, bile ducts, and pancreas, your doctor may combine endoscopy with X-rays in a procedure cleverly named an endoscopic retrograde cholangiopancreatography (ERCP). Following the usual procedure for an endoscopy, dye is injected into the bile ducts so that X-rays can reveal the exact condition of the nearby organs and connective pathways.

Following this procedure, inflammation of the pancreas is not uncommon, but other negative reactions are rare.

Ambulatory esophageal pH study

When there is a need to measure the amount of acid reflux that occurs in a patient, they might perform an ambulatory esophageal pH study. In a procedure similar to an endoscopy, a fine plastic tube is inserted into the GIT, but this time through the nose, where it comes out and is taped to the face, hooked around the ear and attached to a small recorder that looks a bit like a Walkman.

The patient wears this apparatus for twenty-four hours, recording on the machine when she eats, sleeps, etc. This will yield a very exact picture of the changing levels of acidity, and will therefore help to determine treatment. Obviously this is a rather awkward and uncomfortable test and is only performed when an endoscopy won't deliver enough information.

Breath test for *Helicobacter pylori*

In some cases where stomach ulcers are suspected your GP might suggest a breath test rather than an endoscopy. This involves fasting before being given a drink with a solution of urea and a tiny amount of radiation. Half an hour later a breath sample is collected and will indicate the presence or not of *Helicobacter pylori*.

Barium X-rays

Barium X-rays are not used nearly as often as they used to be because endoscopies tell us everything we need to know and more, but in some cases an endoscopy is unavailable.

For what's called an upper GI (gastrointestinal) series, designed to diagnose problems in the esophagus, stomach, and duodenum, the patient drinks a tasteless solution of barium sulphate (thick like a milkshake but not as nice), which is impenetrable by X-rays. The X-rays are taken half an hour after drinking this and will show the outlines of the GIT as opaque white. Although the barium solution is fairly yucky, the procedure isn't uncomfortable.

A radiologist will be able to see ulcers, scar tissue, abnormal growths, hernias, or blockages. Using a machine called a fluoroscope the radiologist can also watch the digestive system work as the barium moves through it, to see, for example, whether the muscles that control swallowing are working well.

Later the barium is passed in the stools but it *can* cause constipation so it's good to increase levels of fiber and water for a few days. It will also turn the stools a grayish-white, so don't freak out.

A lower GI Series can help to diagnose problems in the colon and rectum, revealing conditions including abnormal growths, ulcers, polyps, diverticuli, and cancer. The lower GI series is also called a barium enema, and is much less comfortable than the upper GI. In this case, the radiologist puts the barium solution into your colon through the anus, and there will be a feeling of fullness and pressure in the abdomen making you feel like you need to have a bowel movement. But the tube used to inject the barium has a balloon on the end that prevents the liquid from coming out.

The radiologist will take X-rays with you in different positions to get a complete picture of your lower bowel. Afterward, and with great relief, you will be allowed to use the toilet.

Gastroenterology

Gastroenterologists are medical doctors who specialize in disorders of the gastrointestinal tract. If your doctor suspects or wants to eliminate the possibility of you having anything from stomach ulcers to colorectal cancer, he or she will refer you to a gastroenterologist for further testing.

Gastroenterologists will often perform an endoscopy or a colonoscopy to assess your condition. Once they have diagnosed your problem, they will either treat you themselves or refer you to another specialist or back to your GP for further treatment and advice.

Although they are not also specialists in nutrition or alternative therapies, gastroenterologists are highly trained and incredibly knowledgeable about their particular field, and will generally diagnose and treat your condition in a thoroughly competent, if conventional, manner.

Nutritional science

The science of nutrition has progressed by leaps and bounds in the past few decades, with advances in the field of biomolecular science producing solid evidence for "functional" food and models for effective therapeutic diets. What all this means is that much more than ever before, scientific knowledge is available about how food works inside us and what it can do for us in the long run.

Most treatments for digestive disorders will involve some sort of modification to your diet, and your practitioner will be able to offer you advice on how to proceed. But you might also benefit from the input of a nutritionist specifically trained in remedial food therapy. In other words, someone who can help you figure out what to eat to feel better and *stay* well.

Your visit to a nutritionist could give you a whole new way of seeing the world and fueling your body. In doing so, you can be set on a road to optimum health that will be the result of good eating habits and tricks of the trade you'll be able to draw on for the rest of your life. And you can spread the joy by using some of these nutritional tricks on your family.

You don't need a referral to see a nutritionist, and not all healthcare programs will reimburse you for visiting a registered dietician. In any case, it could be the smartest money you ever spent.

Complementary therapies

Disorders of the digestive tract are especially treatable by complementary therapies, whether on their own or in conjunction with conventional medicine. If you're combining therapies, it's important to remember to inform each practitioner of the other treatments you're getting. Some herbs can interact badly with prescription medicine, while they can enhance others.

Naturopathy

Don't just wander into your local health food store and start filling a shopping basket with a boatload of herbs and vitamins and minerals that claim to help your condition. You need to consult a naturopath before you start forking over the big money, both for your own safety and health and also for your bank account.

Like other practitioners, naturopaths will take a medical history and suggest a range of treatments and therapies, taking a strongly holistic approach. In other words, they'll look at all of your symptoms as well as your general eating habits, stress levels, your body type, and other relevant physical attributes, and not just your digestive condition. The good thing about consulting naturopaths is that they can recommend effective supplements in doses specially tailored to your needs. Usually the recommended dosages on supplement labels refer to daily minimums for a maintenance program and may not be enough to do you any good.

They might also mix up a combination of herbs that will treat your condition in a very individual way. Or they may offer nutritional advice. In any case, remember to be as open with your naturopath as you are with your medical doctor. Being shy never solved anybody's health problems. If a naturopath can't help you, or they need more diagnostic information from blood tests or ultrasounds, they'll refer you to the appropriate medical doctor.

Homeopathy

Homeopathy is practiced worldwide, and has long been popular among diverse groups of people, including Britain's royal family, among others not normally associated with alternative medicine. People who have had their diseases cured swear by their lives on it, and many turn to it before any other kind of medical treatment. But does it work?

Recent studies are inconclusive. Skeptics argue that the supposedly active ingredients in homeopathic medicine are so diluted as to be nonexistent, so there is no possible way the solution (generally taken orally in drops under the tongue) can have any but the placebo effect. Advocates of homeopathy say, "Why then do infants and animals get better when treated this way?"

Unfortunately you will not find a definitive answer here, although a recent report suggests that the idea of "memory of water," which is basic to homeopathy, is a real thing. Hopefully science will soon be able to explain the supposed mechanism involved. In any case, many people with digestive disorders claim to feel the benefits of homeopathic treatment.

As with all remedial disciplines, the effectiveness of homeopathy depends on the skill of the individual practitioner. What good homeopaths do is listen carefully to the description of your symptoms as well as your emotional state, and then suggest a particular remedy. Once you start taking it you should notice an improvement within a day or two. If not, you're on the wrong remedy and you should stop.

Part of the appeal of homeopathic medicine is that it is safe, nonaddictive, fast-working, and cheap (we're sure that's why Queen Elizabeth uses it). But don't expect to be healed by taking an off-the-shelf remedy you buy at the health food store that seems to address your symptoms. The right remedy will more likely be found by a trained professional who will ask questions you wouldn't even have thought to ask.

Osteopathy and chiropractic

Sometimes, structural flaws or dysfunction can contribute to digestive disorders, and practitioners trained in the correction of these can help you find instant relief.

Most people associate osteopathy with the treatment of back pain, but the practice of visceral osteopathy is also common and some osteopaths even specialize in the field.

If you visit an osteopath, they will take a detailed medical history and enquire about your current symptoms. Then they will do a physical examination followed by treatment with gentle hands-on manipulation.

Osteopaths can treat a wide range of gastrointestinal disorders, including indigestion, bloating, hiatus hernias, colic, and IBS, among others. They can even relieve lymphatic congestion by doing gentle manipulation of the throat. Osteopaths will also address problems that arise from the neural link between the spine and the digestive organs, which can become restricted through a variety of things from obesity to bad posture to an accident. Sometimes it just takes one visit to a qualified osteopath and months of discomfort can evaporate.

Chiropractors do less direct visceral work than osteopaths, but many treat hiatus hernias, and they will all address spinal issues that may have an effect on digestive function.

Acupuncture and traditional Chinese medicine

According to its traditional practitioners, acupuncture is an effective treatment for almost every ailment we can suffer from because it stimulates the mind to heal the body by balancing the yin and yang energy flow. It's so successful as a way to block pain that acupuncture is commonly used in China as the primary anesthetic during major surgery. Although acupuncture is now embraced by much of the Western medical establishment as a way to block both acute and chronic pain, many doctors are skeptical about its ability to affect other systems, such as digestion. But many people with digestive disorders have been helped by this ancient Chinese therapy, especially when it's used in conjunction with change of diet and other treatments.

An acupuncturist will observe and question you regarding your current problem to determine the exact nature of your disharmony. So even if you go in complaining about your bowel, you'll be asked about lifestyle, diet, circulation, sleep patterns, and your emotional state. As acupuncture is just part of the practice of traditional Chinese medicine (TCM), you will also have your tongue examined and your pulse felt. The quality, strength, and rhythm of your pulse will reveal *a lot* to a TCM practitioner, who will decide on treatment accordingly.

According to TCM, the practitioner can also tell many things from your tongue, the state of which is completely determined by your digestive health. A person with a perfectly healthy digestive tract will have a nice, flat, pink tongue, but a person with digestive trouble may have a tongue that is white all over, blotchy white with a red rim, swollen, or yellowish. These signs might indicate gastrointestinal toxins, unabsorbed nutrients, too much mucous in the GIT, and even mineral deficiencies. Obviously changes in diet will need to be implemented, but the acupuncturist can also use the needles to stimulate your body's energy to help your organs and systems heal. He or she may also treat you with herbs (fresh or dried) to be used in a tea or simply mixed in a glass of water. This is a very holistic practice!

In ancient times acupuncturists used sharpened stones and, later on, needles carved from bone and bamboo, but now they use sterile steel, gold, or silver needles. The needles are inserted for a second or two, or left in place for up to thirty minutes, depending on your condition. After insertion, the needles are usually rotated.

You *can* get almost immediate results from acupuncture, but it usually takes more than one visit. Often it takes half a dozen visits to really balance your yin and your yang. If you opt for the treatment, don't quit halfway through because you haven't seen results. With this sort of therapy, it takes time. As with most of life's problems, there's no magic bullet.

Ayurvedic medicine

Ayurveda is a Sanskrit word meaning life knowledge, and Ayurvedic medicine is the ancient clinical science of treating the mind, body, and spirit as one integrated organism. Fundamental to Ayurveda is the belief that there are three biological humors, or doshas, that are the pervasive forces of the universe. These humors, called Kapha, Pitta, and Vata, are composed of varying degrees of the five elements: fire, water,

earth, ether, and air. Each of us has a completely unique combination of doshas, and it is this combination that an
Ayurvedic practitioner will try to determine when diagnosing
a problem and recommending a course of action. The key to
good health is balancing the doshas.

Practitioners use a variety of methods to achieve this.
First, they question the patient about emotional and lifestyle
issues (such as "do you get cold hands and feet in winter?" or
"are you a very loyal person?"), then they examine the pulse,
tongue, eyes, nails, and then they check other organs and functions, including the heart, lungs and intestines. Finally, they
will suggest a range of treatments that usually include adjust-
ments to the diet, lifestyle, and certainly emotion and stress
management.

There is even an Ayurvedic restaurant in London where a
physician will assess your health and then recommend what to
order from the menu. People who have suffered chronic digestive trouble have reported feeling good for the first time after
a meal when they eat there.

In any case, Madonna, Demi Moore, and Naomi Camp-
bell have all sung the praises of Aurvedic medicine, and
they've tried everything, so they'd know! With its accent on
dietary and emotional therapy, Ayurvedic medicine seems to
be very effective in dealing with tricky malfunctions of the
gut, especially when conventional medicine has been less than
successful.

Massage and reflexology

It's important to remember how interconnected all of our internal systems are if you want to appreciate how massage can help treat disorders in the gut. Because our digestive organs are connected to the rest of our bodies via a complex network of nerves, blood vessels, and tissues, a good massage that treats those nerves, vessels, and tissues can also treat your stomach, your liver, and your bowel. Sometimes a deep neck massage can release pressure on the vagus nerve, which in turn releases a blockage to the stomach. Many of us have experienced that wonderful gurgling sound in the belly when on the receiving end of a great neck rub.

Reflexology is an incredibly satisfying branch of massage therapy that can also have great therapeutic benefits for the digestive system. The idea is that points of congestion and tension in different parts of the feet and hands mirror congestion and tension in corresponding parts of the body. By stimulating and massaging these points on the feet and hands, the distant affected body parts are stimulated and healed. Chronic constipation is one of the conditions that has been very successfully treated with reflexology. If you have digestive problems and you decide to go for a massage, make sure your therapist also practices reflexology and you are in for a treat.

Colonic irrigation

To many people the idea of lying on a bed while a tube inserted into their rectum pours water into the colon to flush out its contents is bizarre and dangerous. This is not necessarily so. Many people swear by the benefits associated with colonic irrigation, especially as the procedure has become more sophisticated and the facilities are kept at hospital standards of safety and hygiene.

First of all, it's important to describe what it is to dispel the many misconceptions. Essentially, colonic irrigation is a kind of really thorough enema designed to cleanse the colon. What happens is that a trained colonic therapist (a registered nurse if you go to the right place) will insert a thin (thinner than your pinky finger) sterile tube a few centimeters into the rectum. The tube is then attached to a hose that is connected to a container of body temperature water, which flows through the tube with the help of gravity. No extra mechanical pressure is exerted, so there's no chance of perforation as there was in the past. While all this is going on, the person having the colonic irrigation is lying on a comfortable bed with the bottom part cut out and falling away into a built-in toilet bowl.

What generally happens is that a surprising amount of waste matter is eliminated over the course of about an hour. This is mostly a fairly comfortable procedure, but there may be some cramping and nausea that pass pretty quickly.

The theory behind all this is that people with a variety of bowel dysfunctions—from mild to severe—often have a buildup of fecal matter, which can cause everything from bad breath to fatigue to constipation, bloating, and flatulence. Whatever the case, having the colon cleansed of backed-up waste does help it do its job more efficiently, so that after a treatment, or a series of treatments, colonic muscle tone improves and normal peristalsis can resume.

It's essential to repopulate your colon with probiotics after colonic irrigation, as the friendly flora will have been flushed out along with the unfriendly bacteria. People who fail to do this after a colonic treatment risk coming away with worse problems than they went in with.

Colonic irrigation is *not* recommended for children, and anyone with chronic disorders or recent illnesses should check with their doctor before taking the plunge.

If you do decide to try colonic irrigation, make sure you go to a reputable clinic where the staff is trained and the facilities are clean. Some clinics will offer a wide range of intestinal health programs and advice, and can be enormously helpful for people who have tried other therapies and found them lacking. Some alternative practitioners and even medical doctors and oncologists have turned to the use of coffee enemas for the relief of the pain caused by liver and colorectal cancer. Obviously if you have a serious medical condition like cancer, any treatment should be discussed with your doctor and all the aspects of the therapy considered beforehand.

Fasting and detoxification

Our bodies have their own detoxing capabilities, and in perfectly healthy people with excellent diets these are usually enough to keep their internal house clean. But many alternative practitioners believe that every once in a while some of us need a little extra help cleaning house. Chemicals, drugs, environmental pollutants, poor diet, intestinal infections as well as the by-products of natural metabolism can all contribute to stress on the liver, kidneys, and GIT. Many therapists suggest that symptoms of this stress can include constipation, bloating, excessive flatulence, headaches, irritability, joint pain, sweating, nausea, and even palpitations.

Most conventional medical practitioners, as well as many complementary therapists, believe that this whole idea of internal toxic buildup is a gross exaggeration and has filled the pockets of scaremongers who prey on the public's insecurities about their bad habits. But the interesting thing is that most people *do* feel better after "detoxing." But they may merely be experiencing the benefits of cutting out crap from their diets, getting more nutrients from better foods and drinking more water. Whether they unloaded a significant amount of "toxins" is highly debatable.

The important thing is to understand that no detox or fasting program should be undertaken without supervision by a doctor or other health practitioner. A lot of people go off full of high hopes and great expectations on a program that could seriously compromise their health. They read a book and figure they know everything they need to know. But they don't. For example, people with stomach or duodenal ulcers should *never* fast, nor should those undergoing radiation or chemotherapy, or indeed *any* cancer sufferers. People with chronic stomach pain shouldn't fast, and both fasting and any kind of detox program should be off-limits to children, pregnant women, people recovering from surgery, or anyone with ulcerative colitis, Crohn's disease, or diabetes. Many medical conditions and prescription medicine will not interact well with fasting or extreme detoxification diets, so you should always proceed with caution and with the advice of a professional.

That said, both detoxification and fasting programs can work wonders, especially for people who have been suffering with certain digestive disorders for a long time and have tried everything else. There are many different kinds of programs and you should help your practitioner pick the one that's right for your needs and your personality. Some programs last for three days and some for three months or more. You want to do something that you can manage, taking into consideration your health, your lifestyle, your wallet, and your willpower.

Detoxification programs involve restrictive diets where you can eat food, but only certain kinds of food. Once again, the types of restrictions depend on your condition, but usually they will involve abstinence from all fried foods, saturated fats, fatty meats, sugars, alcohol, coffee, black tea, and often foods with additives and preservatives. They may also recommend that you avoid foods high in amines and salicylates, so that white rice is okay but not wild rice, buckwheat flour is good but not corn flour, green beans are cool but not carrots. It all depends what sort of program you and your practitioner have selected. It may also be recommended that you take special vitamin, mineral, or herbal supplements to compensate for what you're giving up and also to help your liver cope with the transition.

The effects of detox diets can usually be felt within a few days. At first you may feel quite sick. Symptoms of detoxing through diet often resemble those experienced by drug addicts going through withdrawal: you may experience nausea, headaches, severe irritability, insomnia, chills, sweats, and possibly even vomiting. Withdrawing from coffee, alcohol, sugar, and other substances we rely on too much can be extremely unpleasant. This will make you *very* grumpy. It's important that loved ones are warned about what you're going through, as this stage has been known to challenge the sturdiest relationships. Usually this stage passes after a few days.

It's also really important to exercise while you're detoxing, as this will help you recover faster, especially if you break a sweat. And remember to drink lots of water to aid the rejuvenation of your liver, kidneys, and GIT. Herbal teas and lemon added to your water will help you get through this ordeal as well.

Massage can also accelerate the process and of course ease your mental and physical suffering as you recover from years of coffee and beer drinking, cigarette smoking, and fast food munching.

The great thing is that when you finish a detox program, you will feel fabulous. So enjoy it for a while and try not to *retox* right away. Your practitioner will continue to guide you through this part of the program, but it's really important to reintroduce foods and other substances gradually if at all. What's nice about this process is that you can really see which individual foods or food accessories disagree with you and your newly pristine digestive system.

Fasting does many of the same things that a detox program will do, but through more extreme methods. In other words, without solid food. Which does *not* mean that you're supposed to starve yourself. Good fasting programs usually involve drinking herbal teas, mineral waters, and vegetable and fruit juices that will not only nourish you but also *supposedly* help flush the toxins out of your body. Once again—sorry to be such a nag—it's vital that fasting be done with the participation of your doctor or other practitioner, such as a nutritionist, naturopath, or herbalist. Fasting isn't for everybody, and each person who undertakes a fast will have different needs. So proceed with extreme caution.

But the good news is that fasting can do all the things detoxing can do—and more. Often stomach disorders such as heartburn, parasitic infections, general bowel laziness, and bad breath can be eliminated with a good fast. But you need to be aware of what your body is going through. After the first day or two your tongue might swell up and your breath might get even worse than it was. Don't be alarmed—this is just part of the fasting experience.

Just like with detoxing, it will help if you exercise while fasting. The increased circulation aids recovery and certainly keeps your mood up. Also, because your body's energy stores aren't busy with digestion, they're more readily available for other activities. People who are on fasts are often amazed at how much energy they have for both physical and mental tasks. Up to a point. Fasting is definitely a relatively short-term proposition, and your condition should be monitored throughout to make sure you're not fading away.

After either a detoxification program or a fast, it's important to replenish your intestines with probiotics, as a lot will have been shed as you cleaned house. Especially after fasting, you might need to jump-start your colon with natural laxatives like prunes or psyllium husks, so have them standing by.

Although many medical doctors and gastroenterologists question the need for detoxification, conventional medicine has often failed to deliver solutions to long-standing problems, so it's worth considering. And if you do it right, and your program is followed under supervision, it certainly can't hurt.

Seven
Exercising for Digestion

Y ou've heard it before, but you'll hear it again: exercise is good for digestion. But is any particular kind better than another? Well, all safe exercise is good for digestion because anything that increases circulation, muscle activity, and deep breathing is going to help you move food along (and out) and absorb nutrients. But certain types of exercise are especially beneficial.

Walking and running

Walking and running are good, because they work *with* gravity to keep acid where it should be (in the stomach) and food continually gets propelled downward. Of course it's not good to exercise right after eating a big meal, as this can cause stitches, nausea, and indigestion. It's important to move around *a little* after eating, but not with vigorous exercise. If you can manage it without keeling over from hunger, it can be good to exercise before breakfast because it stimulates the visceral muscles and helps with that first bowel movement.

Yoga

One of the nicest things you can do for your gut as well as the rest of your body and mind is yoga because it's such a holistic form of exercise. It tones, strengthens, and stretches both your outer musculature and your internal organs while also helping you manage stress, so it's a wonderfully integrated workout especially relative to digestion.

There are several different kinds of yoga, the main ones being Iyengar and Ashtanga. The former involves holding the poses for a long time in order to bring the body and mind into balance, while the latter uses continuous movement and breathing during which you can really work up a sweat. The latest yoga fad is Bikram, where the room temperature is kept at 98.6°F to aid in the loosening of muscles and the release of toxins through the skin.

Which type of yoga you do depends on your own needs, tastes, and the advice of your health professional. Like all forms of exercise, you shouldn't undertake a yoga course unless you're advised that it's safe for you. Some yoga positions can actually exacerbate digestive disorders, so you really need to talk it through before you start. Also, some yoga isn't recommended to women in the first three months of pregnancy, and some poses (like upside-down ones) should be avoided before your period. And make sure you don't eat just before doing yoga. If you try this, you'll quickly discover why it's a bad idea!

When you're starting out, it's best to be part of a yoga class. Coordinating the stretches, poses, and breathing can be tricky at first so it's best to be guided by a teacher.

Pilates

Pilates is one of the best exercises for promoting core stability, that is, the muscles in the deep center of our torsos that maintain balance and strength. And the good news is that toning these very same muscles can help the digestive process.

One of the nice things about Pilates is that it's based on the quality rather than quantity of your exercise. You'll be encouraged to concentrate on each incremental movement and coordinate it precisely with your breathing. This means that anyone at any level of fitness can benefit from Pilates.

If you do a Pilates class, you may use the traditional equipment, such as the universal reformer, which involves a series of springs and weights to help you perform the exercises. Or you may just perform mat work, or floor exercises, where the instructor guides you through a conventional Pilates workout using the weight of your own body. Or you may use the big inflated ball, which is such an incredibly fun and useful way to get the most out of the movements. Whatever the method, Pilates exercises will help you tone and stretch muscles you didn't even know you had, and they are very often the deep, abdominal, and oblique muscles that are intimately bound to your intestinal system. If you become a Pilates fanatic—as so many of us do who try it once and fall in love—your gut will thank you for it.

Abdominal workouts

Any exercise that involves the abdominal muscles will aid digestion. Engaging the abdominals during sit-ups, crunches, or stationary contractions actually massages the bowel, helping to keep it toned and move things along.

If you want to help things along even more, you can gently massage your abdomen in the direction your bowel moves, i.e. up the right side, across your belly button from right to left, and down the left side. After you do this gently, breath deeply, relax, and then repeat. This can be very effective, especially combined with some sit-ups or another abdominal workout.

Eight
The Bottom Line

From top to bottom, from mouth to motion, your digestive health is in your hands. We know so much more than we used to know that there are no more excuses for not addressing what ails you, whether it's reflux or bloating or more serious conditions. And when there are so many different styles of treatment and diet options there's no reason to just put up with indigestion or constipation or bad breath for the rest of your life.

But even if you're not suffering with any chronic condition right now, you may be on the road to digestive hell if you eat and drink the wrong stuff most of the time. And the older you get, the higher the price you'll pay for a diet with too few fruits and vegetables and a lifestyle with too little physical activity. On the other hand, if you eat right most of the time and get some exercise a few times a week, the older you get the longer you'll enjoy the benefits of a happy digestive system.

In some cases, no matter what you do, disease can strike you down. But with healthy eating and regular exercise you're giving yourself the best chance of cheating both mild and serious diseases out of a win. So make yourself the winner. Lightly grill some salmon and steam some vegetables for dinner, and enjoy them along with a glass or two of wine. You deserve it.

Acknowledgments

O ne author alone does not a book make, and *Get to Know Your Gut* would not exist without the talents and enthusiasm of many people. As always, thanks to Jill Brown, smart and stylish commissioning editor at ABC Books in Australia for her input and guidance, and publisher Stuart Neal for his ongoing support of the idea of healthcare books written from the patient's point of view. Also, thanks to Sue McCloskey at Marlowe & Company for recognizing that Americans need help with their guts too!

Also, thanks to Mignon Turpin, Ingo Voss, and Cheryl Rose for contributing to the production of such a user-friendly little tome. Special thanks to the many healthcare practitioners who helped me with various digestive ailments over the years, including Marilyn Golden, Victoria Sutton, Terry Bolin, Gillian Deakin, Peter Edwards, and Bianca James. I learned something useful from every one of them. A huge debt of gratitude also to Joanna McMillan-Price, an astute and enthusiastic consultant and expert on everything to do with food, whom I was incredibly lucky to get as my consultant on the book. Finally, thanks as always to my agent, Deb Callaghan, for her love and support.

Index

A

abdominal workouts, 186-88
acidophilus. *See* probiotics
acid reflux. *See* heartburn
acid suppressants, 137-38
acupuncture, 171-73
acute allergic reactions, 63
AIDS, 88, 145
air, swallowing, 16-17, 89
alcohol, 11, 60, 109-12
alginate, 140
allergens, body's defense against, 13-14
allergies, 31, 62-63
aloe vera (juice or capsules), 21, 58, 98
ambulatory esophageal pH study, 163
American Cancer Society slogan, xiv
amines, 180
anaphylactic shock, 63
anorexia, 92
antacids, over-the-counter, 21, 33, 87, 137-38
antibiotics

candida-related complex from, 79-80
digestion and, 136-37
E. coli, contraindicated for, 40
for inflammatory bowel disease, 72
for ulcers, 60
anti-candida diet, 81-82
antidepressants, 142
anti-diarrhea drugs, 40
anti-inflammatories, 141
antioxidants for colorectal cancer, 86
antispasmodics, 57, 138-39
appendicitis, 73-74
apples as digestive aid, 98
aromatherapy, 152-53
artificial sweeteners, 108-9
Ashtanga yoga, 185
aspartame, 109
aspirin, 60, 143
asthma, 69
Atkins diet, 28
Ayurvedic medicine, 173-74
Aztecs, 25-26

B

BAC (Breath Alcohol Content), 111
bacteria. *See also* probiotics
    antibiotics for, 80, 136-37
    body's defense against, 13-14
    diverticulitus from, 74-75
    fiber for, 120
    in foods, 39-41
    garlic for, 100
    gas and, 17, 19
    Mycobacterium avium paratuberculosis, 72
    stomach acid and, 10
    ulcers from, 59-60
    in yogurt, 103-4
bad breath, 28-29
bananas, 99
barbecuing meats, 85, 123
barium X-rays, 164-65
Barrett's esophagus, 34
beans, gas and, 17-19
bifidus. *See* probiotics
Bikram yoga, 185
bile, 12, 23
bilirubin, 23
bloating, 19, 31, 109
blood
    from colorectal cancer, 84
    in stools, 23, 61
    in urine, 25
    in vomit, 37

blood sugar levels, 118
blood tests, 159-60
booze, 11, 60, 109-12
bottle-fed babies, 89
bowel, 12, 56, 79. *See also* colon; small intestine
bowel gas, 16-21
bowel movements. *See also* fecal matter
    coffee and, 107
    constipation (*See* constipation)
    diarrhea (*See* diarrhea)
    exercise and, 185
    fiber and, 49-50, 120
    Hirschsprung's disease, 82-83
    hormone levels and, 51
    laxatives, 53-54, 57, 140-41
    from smoking, 146
    travel and, 52
breast-feeding, colic from, 89
Breath Alcohol Content (BAC), 111
breath fresheners, 28
breath test for *Helicobacter pylori* (Hp), 163
Buddhist monk experiment, 150, 151
bulimia, 37, 92
bulking agents, 53
burping, 17, 31
burping babies, 89

C

cabbage, 99
calcium, 127-28
cancer
  from alcohol consumption, 112
  chemotherapy, 37
  colorectal, 83-86, 112
  esophageal, 34
  meditation for healing, 150
  stomach, 61, 86-87
  ulcers from, 60-61
candida albicans, 78
candida-related complex (CRC), 78,
  79-82
candidiasis, 78
carbonated water, 116
carcinogens from barbecuing, 85, 123
celery, 99
celiac disease (gluten intolerance),
  65-66, 159
champagne, 112
charcoal tablets, 21
chemotherapy, nausea from, 37
chewing, reasons for, 6-7
chewing gum, 7
children, gastroenteritis in, 47.
  See also infants
Chinese food, 11
chiropractic, 171
cholesterol, fiber and, 120

chyme, 12
cigarette consumption, 34, 60, 145-46
citrus, 116
codeine, 139-40
coffee, 105-7
coffee enemas, 177
cold water versus room temperature,
  116
colic, 88-90
colitis, 70-73
colonic irrigation, 176-78
colon (large intestine)
  colitis, 70-73
  fiber's usefulness in, 120
  gas production in, 17-21
  Hirschsprung's disease, 82-83
  overview, 14, 16
  probiotics and, 130, 137
colonoscopy, 161-62
colorectal cancer, 83-86, 112
complementary therapies. *See also*
  treatments
  acupuncture, 171-73
  Ayurvedic medicine, 173-74
  chiropractic, 171
  colonic irrigation, 176-78
  detoxification, 178-81, 182-83
  fasting, 178-80, 181-83
  homeopathy, 169-70
  massage (*See* massage)
  naturopathy, 167-68

osteopathy, 170-71
overview, 167
reflexology, 175
traditional chinese medicine,
    171-73
constipation
    causes, 23, 24, 50-52, 112, 139-40
    diverticulitis from, 75
    overview, 47-49
    preventing, 48-50, 53
    reflexology for, 175
    treating, 23-24, 52-54
    visualization for healing, 149
    water intake and, 23-24
cooking to minimize gas, 18
cortisone, 60, 72
cranio-sacral treatment for colic,
    90
CRC (candida-related complex), 78,
    79-82
Crohn's disease, 57, 60, 70-73, 82
cryptosporidium, 41

D

dairy products. *See also* milk
    colorectal cancer from, 85-86
    food poisoning and, 40, 41, 45
    intolerance to, 64, 67

dehydration, 25. *See also* water, drinking
    enough
dental health, 5, 7-9, 17, 28
dentures, 17
depression, 142, 153-54
detoxification, 178-81, 182-83
diagnostic tests
    for allergies, 63
    ambulatory esophageal pH study, 163
    barium X-rays, 164-65
    blood tests, 159-60
    for candidiasis, 78
    for celiac disease, 66, 159
    for colorectal cancer, 83-84
    endoscopy, 161-62
    fecal occult blood test, 83-84
    for heartburn (reflux), 163
    for *Helicobacter pylori* (Hp), 159, 161,
        163
    for Hirschsprung's disease, 82-83
    for inflammatory bowel disease, 72
    for irritable bowel syndrome, 57
    for lactose intolerance, 65
    for leaky gut syndrome, 91
    overview, 158-59
    for pancreas, 160, 162
    for stomach cancer, 87
    for ulcers, 59-60
    ultrasound, 160
diarrhea

AIDS and, 88
from alcohol overindulgence, 112
as bowel's inability to absorb water, 24
in children, 47
fiber for, 120
as symptom of food poisoning, 40
treating, 45, 138-40
diet. *See also entries beginning with* food
after food poisoning episode, 45-46
anti-candida, 81-82
colorectal cancer and, 85-86
feeling of hunger, 11-12
fiber, amount of, 118
food allergies, 31, 62-63
food intolerance, 29, 31, 62, 64-66
gallbladder disease and, 77
gas and, 17-21
for indigestion, 98-104
inflammatory bowel disease and, 72-73
irritable bowel syndrome and, 58, 72-73
overindulgence, 67-68
"Western," 69-70, 71-72
dietary versus functional fiber, 118
digestion, foods that aid, 98-104
digestion of meat, 122-23
digestive aid tables, 31, 44, 70
digestive disorders. *See also* gas

anorexia, 92
appendicitis, 73-74
bulimia, 92
candida, 78-82
colic, 88-90
colitis, 70-73
colorectal cancer, 83-86, 112
constipation (*See* constipation)
Crohn's disease, 57, 60, 70-73, 82
diarrhea (*See* diarrhea)
diverticulitis, 74-75
food allergies, 31, 62-63
food intolerance, 29, 31, 62, 64-66
food sensitivities (*See* food sensitivities)
gall bladder disease, 23, 76-78, 160
gastroenteritis, 38-39
halitosis, 28-29
heartburn, 30-35, 98-104
hemorrhoids, 54-55
hiatus hernia, 33, 90-91
hormonal fluctuations, 91-92 (*See also* hormones)
indigestion, 30-35, 98-104
inflammatory bowel disease, 70-73
irritable bowel syndrome, 56-59, 72-73, 79, 142
leaky gut syndrome, 65, 91
nausea, 35-38, 100-101
overview, 27

reasons for, xiii-xiv
reflux, 30-35, 98-104
stomach cancer, 61, 86-87
stomach ulcers (*See* stomach ulcers)
support groups for, 93
ulcerative colitis, 70-73
vomiting, 35-38, 45, 100-101
digestive enzymes. *See* enzymes
digestive enzyme supplements, 126-27
digestive juices
alcoholic stimulation of, 110
chewing food and, 6-7
chewing gum and, 7
sensory stimulation and, 4-5
stomach and, 10
digestive system
blood supply and, 146
bowel, 12, 56, 79 (*See also* colon; small intestine)
diagram, 3, 18
esophagus, 9-10
food "accessories" and, 105-12
gas, 16-21
overview, 1-4, 190-91
saliva, 5
stomach, 10-12
stools, 22-24
teeth, 7-9
tongue and taste buds, 5-6
diverticulitis, 74-75

doctors. *See* physician, visiting your
drugs (prescription)
acid suppressants, 137-38 (*See also* antacids)
alginate, 140
antibiotics (*See* antibiotics)
antidepressants, 142
anti-diarrhea, 40
anti-inflammatories, 141
antispasmodics, 57, 138-39
fasting and, 179
herbs and, 129
lipase inhibitors, 144
muscle relaxers, 138-39
nonsteroidal anti-inflammatory drugs, 60, 143
opioid analgesics, 139-40
overview, 95-96, 135-36
tranquilizers, 142
duodenum, 12
dysbiosis, 131-32

E

E. coli, 39-40
eating disorders, 92
eating recommendations. *See* diet
eating slowly, 7
electrolytes, 37-38, 45

Endoscopic Retrograde Cholangiopancreatography (ERCP), 162
endoscopy, 60, 161-62
enteroscopy, 161-62
enzymes
  for alcohol metabolism, 110-12
  antibiotics and, 137
  gas and, 19
  for milk intolerance, 64-65
  overview, 126-27
  parasites and, 41
  in stomach "juice," 10
epsom salts, 141
ERCP (Endoscopic Retrograde
  Cholangiopancreatography), 162
esophageal cancer, 34
esophageal sphincter, 9, 30
esophageal valve, 33, 90, 92
esophagitis, 34
esophagus, 9-10, 33-34
essential fatty acids, 99-100
exercise
  abdominal workouts, 186-88
  for colorectal cancer, 86
  for constipation, 50
  detoxing and, 181
  drinking water before, 115
  fasting and, 182
  for healing stress, 155
  overview, 184

Pilates, 186-87
running, 184-85
walking, 184-85
yoga, 185-86

F

farting, 16-19, 109
fasting, 178-80, 181-83
fatty acids, 73, 99-100
fatty foods
  bad breath from, 28-29
  constipation from, 52
  digestion of, 11
  gallstones from, 76
  lipase inhibitors and, 144
fecal matter. *See also* bowel movements
  bulking agents, 49-50, 53
  E. coli from infected, 40
  elimination of, 14, 16
  examining, 83-84
  fermentation of, 19
  overview, 22-24
  softeners, 53, 141
fecal occult blood test (FOBT), 83-84
fecal softener laxatives, 53, 141
fiber
  adding to diet, 19
  AIDS and, 88

for colorectal cancer, 85
for constipation, 49-50
for diverticulosis, 75
fruits and vegetables with, 98-104
gas and, 17-19
overview, 114-15, 118-21
psyllium husks, 49-50
stools and, 23-24
fiber-optic video camera, 161
figs, 100
filtered water, 117
fish, value in diet, 100
flatulence. *See* gas
flatus, 17
flaxseed tea, 101
flossing, 8, 28
fluoroscope, 164
FOBT (fecal occult blood test), 83-84
food
    "accessories," 105-12
    bacteria in, 39-41
    detoxing and re-adding, 180-81
    digestion health from, 98-104
    eating too much of any particular, 69
    fatty (*See* fatty foods)
    as functional, 95, 166
    for healing indigestion, 98-104
    meats, 85, 121-23
    parasites in, 41-42
    versus pharmaceuticals, 95-96

raw, 124
water with, 115-16
welcoming, 97-98
food allergies, 31, 62-63
food elimination, 30, 33
food intolerance, 29, 31, 62, 64-66
food poisoning
    dairy products and, 40, 41, 45
    milk sensitivities from, 67
    overview, 39-42
    preventing, 42-44
    treating, 45-47
food sensitivities
    bad breath from, 29
    from candida-related complex, 78
    low stomach acid and, 31
    overview, 62, 67-70
    during pregnancy, 92
    testing for, 58
friendly flora in gut, 20, 130-34, 137
friends, value of, 154-55
fruits and fruit juices, 19, 47, 116
fruits for indigestion, 98-104
frying meats, 85
functional versus dietary fiber, 118

G

gall bladder, 12

gall bladder disease, 23, 76-78, 160
gallstones, 23, 76
garlic, 100
gas
    from artificial sweeteners, 109
    bloating, 19, 31, 109
    burping, 17, 31
    causes, list of, 20-21
    controlling, 19, 21
    farting, 16-19, 109
    production in colon, 17-21
    from swallowing air, 16-17, 89
gastritis, 110-11
gastroenteritis, 38-39. *See also* digestive
    disorders
gastroenterologists, 57, 161, 165-66
gastrointestinal tract (GIT), 2-4
gastroscopy, 161
genetic predispositions, 64, 65, 84
giardia, 41
ginger, 100-101
GIT (gastrointestinal tract), 2-4
gluten intolerance (celiac disease),
    65-66, 159
grains, over-consumption of, 68
grapefruit, 101
grinding teeth, 8-9
gut, meaning of term, 2

H

halitosis, 28-29
heartburn (reflux)
    diagnostic tests, 163
    foods for healing, 98-104
    overview, 30-35
    from smoking, 145
Helicobacter pylori (Hp)
    diagnostic tests, 159, 161, 163
    overview, 59-60
    stomach cancer and, 87
    wine protects against, 110
hemolytic uremic syndrome, 40
hemorrhoids, 54-55. *See also* constipation
herbal bitters, 70
herbalists, 128-29
herbs and herbal teas
    for constipation, 50
    detoxing and, 181-82
    for food poisoning, 45
    for indigestion, 101-2, 103
    for irritable bowel syndrome, 58
    minimizing gas with, 21
    for morning sickness, 36
    naturopaths and, 168
    overview, 128-29
    pharmaceuticals and, 129
    in traditional chinese medicine,
        172-73

hiatus (hiatal) hernia, 33, 90-91
Hirschsprung's disease, 82-83
HIV/AIDS, 145
holistic approach, 168
homeopathy, 169-70
hormones
    constipation from swings of, 51
    fiber and, 120
    fluctuations in, 91-92
    intestinal ecology and, 80
    relaxin, 30, 51
    stress and, 147-48
    Zollinger-Ellison syndrome, 60
hunger, as "not overfilled" feeling, 11
hydrochloric acid (stomach), 10,
    30-31, 111

I

IBD (inflammatory bowel disease),
    70-73
IBS. *See* irritable bowel syndrome
ibuprofen, 60, 143
ileocecal valve, 14
immune system
    AIDS, 88
    allergies and, 62-63
    candidiasis and, 78
    inflammatory bowel disease and, 71
    intestines and, 13-14

indigestion, 30-35, 98-104
infants. *See also* children
    colic, 88-90
    gastroenteritis in, 46
    Hirschsprung's disease, 82-83
inflammatory bowel disease (IBD),
    70-73
internal bleeding from colorectal
    cancer, 84. *See also* blood
intestinal lining
    candida and, 79
    colorectal cancer in, 84
    fatty acids for maintaining, 100
    fiber and, 120
    role of healthy, 13-14
intestinal tract, overindulgence and,
    69-70
intestines. *See* colon; small intestine
intolerance. *See* food intolerance
iron, 107-8
iron supplements, 125-26
irritable bowel syndrome (IBS)
    cancer and, 58-59
    candida-related complex and, 79
    causes, 56-57
    coffee and, 107
    diagnostic tests, 57
    overview, 55-56
    treating, 57-58, 72-73, 142
Iyengar yoga, 185

J

Japan, 72

K

kidney failure, 40

L

lactase, 64, 67
lactic acid, 104
lactose intolerance, 64, 67, 104
large intestine. *See* colon
laxatives, 53-54, 57, 140-41
leaky gut syndrome, 65, 91
legumes, gas and, 17-19
lemon, 116
licorice tea, 50, 101
lime, 116
linoleic acids, 99-100
linseed tea, 101
lipase inhibitors, 144
liver, 12, 23, 111, 159-60
lower GI Series (barium X-ray),
    164-65
lubricants (for constipation), 53
lymph nodes, 13

M

magnesium for constipation
    prevention, 53
maltitol, 109
mangoes, 101
mannitol "421," 19, 109
MAP (*Mycobacterium avium
    paratuberculosis*), 72
marijuana, 37, 144-45
massage
    for constipation, 52-53, 188
    detoxing and, 181
    for hiatus hernia, 90-91
    overview, 175
meat-eaters, 85, 121-23
medical needs. *See* physician, visiting
    your
medical tests. *See* diagnostic tests
medical treatments. *See* treatments
meditation, 150-51
memory of water, 169
menstruation, yoga and, 186
microvilli, 13
milk. *See also* dairy products
    intolerance to, 64, 67
    Mycobacterium avium paratuberculosis, 72
    raw, 40, 65
mint tea, juice, or sauce, 101-2
miso, 102

morning sickness, 36, 101
morphine, 139-40
motion. *See* bowel movements
motion sickness, 37
mouthwash, 28
mucous in stools, 22-23, 47
muscle relaxers, 138-39
Mycobacterium avium paratuberculosis
  (MAP), 72

N

nausea and vomiting, 35-38, 100-101
nitrates, 106
nonessential fatty acids, 99-100
nonsteroidal anti-inflammatory drugs
  (NSAIDs), 60, 143
NSAIDs (nonsteroidal anti-
  inflammatory drugs), 60, 143
nutrients, 13, 159
nutrition, 66, 158
nutritional science, 166-67

O

oligosaccharides, 130
omega 3 and omega 6, 99-100
opioid analgesics, 139-40

oranges, 102
osteopathy, 170-71
overweight, reflux from, 33-34

P

pancreas, 12, 23, 160, 162
parasites, 41-42, 88, 100
pears, 102
peptic ulcers. *See* stomach ulcers
period, yoga and, 186
peristalsis, 9, 14, 56
peristalsis, reverse, 35
peritonitis, 61, 74
pets, parasites from, 43
pharmaceuticals. *See* drugs
physician, visiting your
  for black stools, 23, 61
  for blood in urine, 25
  for candida-related complex, 81
  chiropractor, 171
  for food poisoning, 46-47
  for gall bladder disease, 77
  gastroenterologist, 57, 161, 165-66
  general recommendation, 29
  for heartburn (reflux), 34-35
  for inadequate digestive enzymes,
    126-27
  for irritable bowel syndrome, 57

for nausea or vomiting, 37
osteopath, 170-71
overview, 156-58
for worms, 42
Pilates, 186-87
plant extracts (aromatherapy), 152-53
polyps, 84
poo-gazing, 84
posture, reflux from, 33-34
post-viral syndrome, 67
prebiotics, 130-34
pregnancy
    constipation during, 51, 91
    heartburn during, 30
    miscarriage from essential oils, 153
    morning sickness, 36
    yoga and, 186
prescriptions. *See* drugs; treatments
preservatives, 106
probiotics (acidophilus and bifidus)
    after detoxing or fasting, 182-83
    after vomiting or diarrhea, 45
    antibiotics killing off, 80
    for candida-related complex, 81
    colonic irrigation and, 177
    for colorectal cancer, 86
    gas reduction with, 21
    for inflammatory bowel disease, 73
    for irritable bowel syndrome, 58

laxative abuse and, 141
overview, 130-34
repopulating intestinal flora with, 130, 137
in yogurt, 103-4
proctoscopy, 161-62
prokinetic drugs, 33
prostaglandins, 143
prunes for constipation, 53, 102
psyllium husks, 49-50
pulse, Traditional Chinese Medicine and, 172
pumpkin, 103
pyloric stenosis, 61
pylorus valve, 12

R

raw food, 124
reflexology, 175
reflux. *See* heartburn
relaxation. *See* stress management
relaxin (hormone), 30, 51
reproductive hormones, 80
running, 184-85

S

saccharine, 109
salicylates, 180
saliva, 4, 5
salmonella, 39
seaweed, 103
senses, digestive process and the, 4-6
sensitivities. *See* food sensitivities
sight, sense of, 4
sigmoidoscopy, 161-62
sleep depravation, 155
slippery elm, 103
small intestine
    Crohn's disease, 57, 60, 70-73, 82
    overview, 12-14, 15
smell, sense of, 4
smoking, 34, 60, 145-46
sorbitol "420," 19, 109
sound, sense of, 4
sparkling water, 116
steroids, 60, 72
stimulant cathartic laxatives, 53, 140
stomach, 10-12, 90-91, 161
stomach acid, 10, 30-31, 111
stomach cancer, 61, 86-87
stomach ulcers
    alcohol and, 111
    coffee and, 107
    from NSAIDs, 143
    overview, 59-61

from smoking, 145
soothing with bananas, 99
from steroids, 60
stools. *See* fecal matter
stool softeners, 53, 141
stress
    constipation from, 50-51
    depression versus, 153-54
    overview, 147-48
    sleep depravation, 155
    symptoms of, 178
stress management
    alcohol for, 110
    aromatherapy, 152-53
    for irritable bowel syndrome, 57
    meditation, 150-51
    overview, 148, 154-55
    visualization, 149-50
sucralose, 109
sugar, 18, 118
supplements. *See also* herbs and herbal
    teas
    calcium, 127-28
    digestive enzymes, 126-27
    overview, 125
    probiotic, 132-33
    vitamins and minerals, 89, 125-26,
        146
support groups, 93
swallowing air, 16-17, 89
symbiotics, 131

symptoms
of appendicitis, 73-74
of candida-related complex, 79
of celiac disease, 65
of colorectal cancer, 86
of diverticulitis, 75
of food sensitivities, 69
of gall bladder disease, 76
of inflammatory bowel disease, 71
of stomach cancer, 87
treating only, 138
of ulcers, 59

T

taste buds, 5-6
TCM (traditional chinese medicine),
   171-73
tea, non-herbal, 107. *See also* herbs and
   herbal teas
teeth, 5, 7-9
tests. *See* diagnostic tests
tetrahydrocannabinol (THC), 145
THC (tetrahydrocannabinol), 145
therapies. *See* complementary
   therapies
throwing up, 35-38, 45, 100-101
tofu, 103
tongue, 5-6, 172
toothpaste, 28

Traditional Chinese Medicine (TCM),
   171-73
tranquilizers, 142, 153-54
travel, constipation from, 51-52
treatments. *See also* complementary
   therapies; drugs; herbs and herbal
   teas
   appendicitis, 74
   celiac disease, 66
   colic, 89-90
   constipation, 23-24, 52-54
   diarrhea, 45, 138-40
   food poisoning, 45-47
   gall bladder disease, 77
   hiatus hernia, 90-91
   indigestion and/or heartburn, 33
   inflammatory bowel disease, 72-73
   irritable bowel syndrome, 57-58,
      142
   lactose intolerance, 64
   reflux, 34
   stomach cancer, 87
   vomiting, 45
tumors, 84

U

ulcerative colitis, 70-73
ulcers. *See* stomach ulcers
ultrasound, 160

upper GI Series (barium X-ray), 164
urine, 25-26, 117

V

vagotomy, 61
vagus nerve, 2-4, 175
vegetables, 98-104, 124
villus, 13
visualization, 149-50
vitamin B deficiency, 89
vitamins and minerals, 89, 125-26,
    146
vomiting, 35-38, 45, 100-101

W

walking, 184-85
waste. *See* fecal matter
water, drinking enough
    for constipation, 48-49
    detoxing and, 181
    with food, 115-16
    overview, 23-26, 113-14,
        115-17
    replacing fluids, 37-38
    traveling and, 44
"Western" diet, 69-70, 71-72
wheat, 65, 66
white blood cells, 13

wine, 110, 112
worms (parasites), 41-42, 100

X

X-rays, 162, 164-65
xylitol, 109

Y

yoga, 185-86
yogurt, 103-4, 127

Z

Zollinger-Ellison syndrome, 60